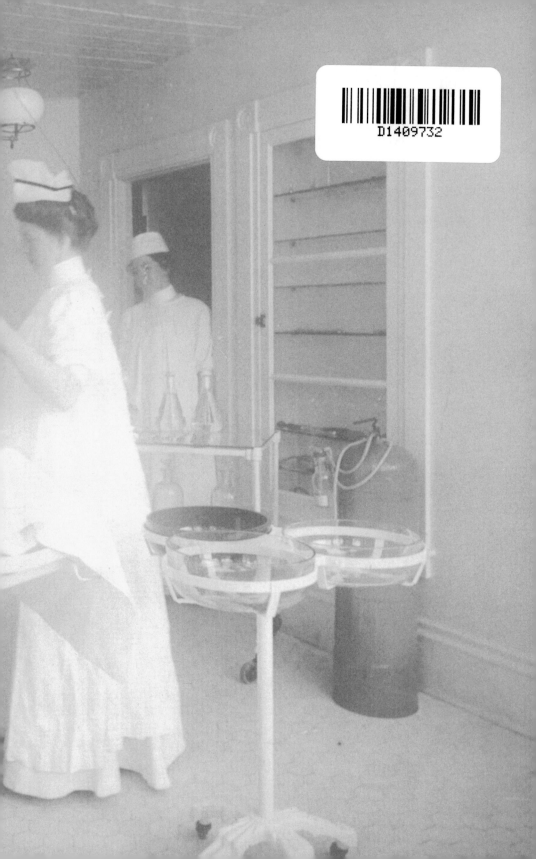

A KINDLY INTEREST

A
KINDLY
INTEREST

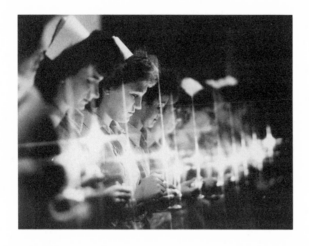

*The Men and Women of Concord Hospital
and Its School of Nursing, 1884 - 1989*

by

Jill C. Wilson

Published for the

CONCORD   HOSPITAL
by
PHOENIX PUBLISHING
West Kennebunk, Maine

Library of Congress Cataloging-in-Publication Data

Wilson, Jill C., 1937-
    A kindly interest: the men and women of Concord Hospi-
tal and its school of nursing, 1884-1989/by Jill C. Wilson.
        p. cm.
    Bibliography: p. 145
    Includes index.
    ISBN 0-914659-41-3
    1. Concord Hospital (Concord, N.H.) — History. 2.
Hospitals — New Hampshire — Concord — History. I. Title.
RA982.C662C69   1989
362.1'1'0974272 — dc19   89-30560
                                                              CIP

Copyright 1989 by Concord Hospital

Printed in the United States of America

CONTENTS

FOREWORD

I had been planning to request permission to write a history of the school of nursing when its phaseout was announced in the fall of 1986. Then, more than ever the idea seemed a good one, for the history could help to ease the closure in the minds of students and faculty, providing a memento of the school's hundred years of educating nurses.

When the project was brought to the attention of Administrator Richard Warner he urged me to include the history of the hospital as well, for none had yet been written. Fortunately, in my opinion then and now, the two could not be separated. The fortunes of the hospital have always affected the life of the school, while periodic shortages of graduate nurses have seriously disturbed the staffing of patient units.

No thought has been given to emphasizing one at the expense of the other. This is a history of people and of events. At times the hospital's concerns were pre-eminent, at other times the needs of the school predominated. I have attempted to relate our hospital and its school to the events of their time, illustrating the context within which change was effected and advances made.

The reader will note that, in health care, progress occurs of late in inverse proportion to the amount of governmental regulation of its activity, a condition that has worked both for and against the patient. Because I imagine that the technical ramifications of the health care regulatory system are as uninteresting to the average reader as they are to me, they do not play a large part in my telling of the story. In fact many of the people who have shaped the history of our institution were and are private citizens unconnected with medicine and nursing, volunteers whose objectives have been "a kindly interest" in the provision of health care to the Concord community.

If one needs an additional reason for a hospital history, consider the following announcement broadcast over the paging system recently: "Will the owner of a blue Chevrolet with license number — please move your car. You are parked on the helipad."

Help with the preparation of this volume has come from many people, all of whom have my deep appreciation. Sheila McCabe guided me to records and scrapbooks in storage. Caroline Antonelli found an additional cache of records and photographs. Elaine Hoyt provided much assistance with school records. Patricia Tobin is largely responsible for many of the photographs and for the graduate lists compiled over the past two years with the help of alumnae, especially former faculty member Helen Love. My son Andrew Wilson helped drag me into the computer age. I am grateful to Elaine Hoyt, Kay Yeaple, and Richard Warner for reading the manuscript and to my husband Bob for his encouragement.

Jill C. Wilson

Concord, New Hampshire
December 1, 1988

A
KINDLY
INTEREST

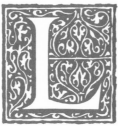*adies and gentlemen . . . as*

you go out from here to your

several duties, I trust you will all

keep alive a kindly interest for

the Margaret Pillsbury Hospital

and its donors.

The statement above from which the title of this volume is derived was made by Dr. Ferdinand Stillings in closing the ceremonies dedicating the Margaret Pillsbury General Hospital in October 1891, a noteworthy event in the evolution of the Concord Hospital and its School of Nursing.

A Chronology of Events

1751   The first United States hospital founded in Philadelphia.

1791   Incorporation of the New Hampshire Medical Society.

1812   Concord Female Charitable Society founded by Elizabeth McFarland.

1842   New Hampshire Asylum for the Insane opened in Concord.

1849   Elizabeth Blackwell graduated from Geneva Medical College.

1856   Crimean War ended, marking establishment of modern nursing by Florence Nightingale.

1868   American Medical Association advocated formal training for nurses.

1873   Bellevue, Connecticut, and Boston training schools for nurses founded.

1884   Concord Hospital Association incorporated-opened first general hospital in New Hampshire at corner Allison and Turnpike Streets.

1888   New Hampshire Asylum for the Insane opened training school.

1889   Concord Hospital Association inaugurated training school.

1891   Margaret Pillsbury General Hospital dedicated on South Main Street.

1896   New Hampshire Memorial Hospital for Women and Children opened on South Spring Street

1897   New Hampshire Memorial Hospital training school opened.

1924   New Hampshire Memorial opened South Spring Street building.

1946   New Hampshire Memorial and Margaret Pillsbury Hospitals merged to form Concord Hospital.

1950   The Alumnae Association of the Concord Hospital incorporated.

1956   Concord Hospital opened at 250 Pleasant Street.

1

1962   *Concord Hospital School of Nursing moved into its own building adjacent to hospital.*

1973   *Concord Hospital expanded and remodelled building, raising bed capacity from 195 to 232.*

1983   *Hospital built major addition, expanding to 295 beds.*

1985   *Concord Hospital reorganized corporate structure.*

1989   *Medical office building opened on hospital campus.*

1989   *Concord Hospital School of Nursing graduated last class.*

2

1

Concord

A Hundred Years Ago

---

merging from the quiet antiquity of the New Hampshire Historical Society's library, the historian re-enters the late twentieth century of a bustling New England capital city, or so it would seem. For Concord, in the summer of 1884, when twenty men and women gathered to discuss establishing a hospital, bustled then, too. It was an exceptionally busy railroad and commercial hub, not the sedate backwater we envision of the 1880s. True, there were only 14,000 people in the city then, half the number here a hundred years later, but the level of sophistication in New Hampshire's capital was high indeed.

The nationally acclaimed humorist, Josh Billings, was delighting audiences in January at White's Opera House. Buffalo Bill appeared later in the year, and the local critic, writing in the *Concord Monitor* disdained a travelling production of *Uncle Tom's Cabin*: "The play was cut until Mrs. Stowe herself never would recognize it and the actors ranted and strutted like the veriest of novices. . . . As usual in the Uncle Tom companies of late years, the best acting was done by the four-footed jackass. We say four-footed to distinguish him from the rest of the company."[1]

William B. Durgin received congratulations on the growth and quality of his small silver-manufacturing business. In 1912 one of his designers would produce the Fairfax pattern, to become the largest selling flatware pattern ever, still on tables across the country today.[2]

Abbot and Downing coaches, Prescott pianos, organs and bass viols, granite from the several quarries near the city, and the many ingenious inventions

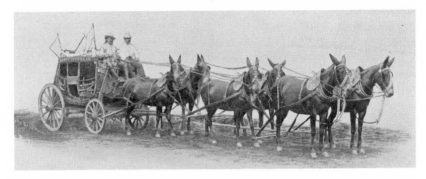

Colonel William F. (Buffalo Bill) Cody in the celebrated Deadwood Coach built in 1863 by the Abbot-Downing Company. It returned to Concord in 1895 for a July 4 appearance still bearing its original wheels.

of the nearby Shakers were other products to spread the fame of Concord, while the printing industry circulated it in books, periodicals and sheet music.

Young Willard Scudder was earning the prize for the best paper on *Macbeth* at fashionable St. Paul's School in Millville outside the city, where he later became a much-loved master. That winter a grieving couple arrived on the train to carry back to Cincinnati the body of their son, killed in a sledding accident near the school.

A new passenger station for the Concord Railroad was enthusiastically described in the *Monitor*. Designed by B.S. Gilbert of New York City, it was to be the last word in luxurious convenience for passengers leaving or arriving on one of the fifty or so daily trains passing through the city.

Progressive whist parties, afternoon teas, chafing dish parties, musicales, receptions, luncheons, and club meetings were described as popular activities of Concord women by Frances Abbott, writing in Lyford's *History of Concord*, published in 1903. Miss Abbott had graduated from Vassar College in 1881, the first Concord girl to take the baccalaureate degree, and she contributed to many of the popular periodicals of the day. Women were active in the life of the city; Mary Parker Woodworth became the first woman to serve on the Board of Education in 1890. Grace Blanchard, the first woman to hold municipal office, was appointed city librarian in 1895. Miss Abbott tells us that in 1896 Concord boasted thirty-nine women's clubs, including ten devoted to the study of Shakespeare which had their own room in the Fowler Library, probably the only room of its kind in the United States.[3]

Nationally, Chester Arthur was in the White House, if briefly, having served from the day James A. Garfield was assassinated until the inauguration of Grover Cleveland, forty-one and a-half months later in March 1885. Earlier in 1884 Theodore Roosevelt had lost his young wife to Bright's disease, the same ailment said to cause the death at fifty-six, of the poet Emily Dickinson just two years later.[4]

And so we are drawn to the subject of health care in the Victorian period, particularly in New England.

Benjamin Franklin had supported the establishment of the country's first hospital in Philadelphia, but even earlier, in 1726 a Dr. Henry Rolfe had spent a winter in Concord, leaving in the spring, never to be heard from again. Concord's first active physician arrived a few years later when the population was 250, and he practiced here for 27 years. Dr. Philip Carrigain followed him and in 1791 the legislature incorporated the New Hampshire Medical Society.[5]

In 1848, after a year of travel throughout the country to observe the deplorable conditions in asylums, Dorothea Dix appealed to Congress for aid to mental patients. Franklin Pierce (the only United States president from New Hampshire) vetoed the resulting bill, believing it the states' duty to provide for the mentally ill.[6] By this time the New Hampshire Asylum for the Insane had been in existence in Concord for six years, incidentally, opening in the same year that the railroad arrived in the city. We know that Concord's first woman physician, Martha J. Flanders, came here to practice with Dr. Alpheus Morrill who was most interested in encouraging women to study medicine. Dr. Flanders was here from 1861 to 1863 when she left to settle in Lynn, Massachusetts. As for nursing, an article in *New England Magazine* for June 1895 has identified Harriet Patience Dame as "perhaps Concord's most valuable contribution to the Civil War." She was an army nurse, presumably without formal training, who served for four years and eight months caring for soldiers of the Second New Hampshire Volunteers, not in a hospital but on the battlefield, distinguishing herself for bravery as well as her nursing skills.

The Crimean War in which Britain, France, and Turkey fought Russia for control of access to the Mediterranean from the Black Sea, began in 1854. By its conclusion in 1856 modern nursing had been born in Britain, the legendary Florence Nightingale its creator. Without detailing her truly heroic effort in bringing about order, cleanliness, and health to the Barrack Hospital at Scutari, and lowering the mortality rate of the British soldiers from 60 percent to 1 percent amidst great opposition from army physicians, it is fair to say that no other individual in the history of nursing has had so great an impact on the profession.[7]

Of major importance to nursing history is her role in establishing the first training school for nurses in London upon her return from Crimea. Armed with funds totalling more than $220,000 contributed by the British public, Florence Nightingale founded a training school at St. Thomas's Hospital, again with great opposition from London physicians. Though so weakened by her own bout with Crimean fever that she never actually supervised her school, Miss Nightingale was its chief advisor. She communicated with the public largely through her writing. *Notes on Matters Affecting the Health, Efficiency and Hospital Administration of the British Army*(1858), and *Notes on Hospitals*(1859), were well received, but it is her *Notes on Nursing*(1859), which served for many years as the definitive text on nursing and is today frequently quoted in texts and articles on the profession, and always quoted at nursing school graduations.[8]

By 1873 when the first hospital census was taken in America there were 178 institutions. Presumably women physicians were attending patients in some of them inasmuch as back in 1849 Elizabeth Blackwell, a graduate of Geneva Medical College, had become the first woman to practice medicine. Nursing, however, remained in a primitive state. As Susan Reverby states in an article based on her book, *Ordered to Care: the Dilemma of American Nursing*, " . . . nursing did not appear de novo at the end of the nineteenth century. As with most medical and health care, nursing throughout the Colonial era and most of the nineteenth century took place within the family and the home."[9] She describes the role of "duty" in women's caring for family members and friends, a role which enlarges as the century progresses with an expanding economy affecting women of various social classes in different ways. While an upper class woman might become active in one or more of the increasingly institutionalized charitable organizations, a working class woman who had had experience at home in nursing a husband or employer might then seek formal employment as a nurse. It was these women, trained only by experience in a home setting, who provided care in America's new hospitals. Reverby tells of Eliza Higgins, matron of Boston's Lying-In Hospital in 1875, who could not find an extra nurse to cover all the deliveries. "In desperation she moved the hospital laundress up to the nursing position, while a recovering patient took over the wash." Little wonder then that there was a great deal of interest in improving the situation, not yet to create a degree of professionalism, but simply to better care for patients in this new hospital setting.[10]

The first American training school for nurses was organized in Boston at the New England Hospital for Women and Children which was staffed by women physicians. Dr. Marie Zakrzewska, who arrived in 1859, suggested practical instruction in the hospital for women medical students and that a school of nursing be established. On September first a class of five students commenced the one year course. Dr. Susan Dimock, coming from studies in Kaiserwerth, Germany, where Florence Nightingale had trained, administered the school. The work was so rigorous that only one student graduated: Melinda Ann (Linda) Richards, who has been called America's first trained nurse.[11]

The year 1873 was perhaps a watershed in that three of the country's greatest training schools made their debuts within the space of a few months, all based on the English or Nightingale model. New York City's Bellevue Hospital opened in May, followed by the Connecticut Training School in New Haven, and in November, the Boston Training School at Massachusetts General Hospital.[12]

Thus the stage was set for important events in Concord beginning on July 3, 1884, which culminated in the Concord Hospital Association, shortly thereafter to become the Margaret Pillsbury Hospital.

2

Benefactors, Beneficiaries

oncord's social conscience is obvious to the newcomer who discovers a range of human services and cultural activities that many a larger community might envy. What is not immediately obvious is that citizens have initiated most of these organizations and energetic volunteer boards have operated them. So it has always been in New Hampshire's capital, whether by virtue of the celebrated Puritan work ethic or simply a recognition that certain needs within the community remain unfunded by legislative act.

For every organization begun in the last twenty years by its citizens, Concord has one which has likely celebrated a hundreth birthday. One of the earliest is the Concord Female Charitable Society founded in 1812 by Mrs. Elizabeth McFarland, wife of the third minister of Old North Church.[1] The mid-1840s brought the Rolfe and Rumford Home, or Asylum, as it was known then. Its benefactor was Sarah Countess of Rumford, daughter of Concord's famous citizen of the world, Benjamin Thompson, Count Rumford. The considerable estate of the countess was left largely to charitable institutions, an early example of such benevolence to future generations.[2]

In the mid-1880s Concord's Flower Mission began surprising less fortunate residents with cheerful bouquets delivered by sympathetic ladies who did not omit the accompanying social call. Periodically members of this group have debated the value of flowers in the face of more serious need, but the flowers prevail while other organizations have come along to provide the necessities of life in a cold New England climate.

Here, as was customary in early days, the sick and elderly were cared for at home, the scene of birth and death. Only the poor and indigent went to hospitals, then usually to die at the hands of the uneducated and unskilled amid the nonexistent sanitation prevalent before the advent of the germ theory.

Influential among American women was Sarah Josepha Hale, editor of the country's most popular women's magazine. *Godey's Lady's Book* gave advice to homemakers on every aspect of the gracious life but Mrs. Hale was a practical person, publishing discussions on the diagnosis and treatment of the common ills of the day. A woman of vision as well, in 1871 she wrote a significant editorial calling for the elevation of the sick nurse to " . . . a profession which an educated lady might adopt without a sense of degradation either on her own part or in the estimation of others. . . . There can be no doubt that the duties of sick nurse, to be properly performed, require an education and training little if at all, inferior to those possessed by members of the medical profession. . . . "[3] She advocated a course of training especially for the nurse with its own body of knowledge culminating in a degree and a diploma. Hospitals began to take her advice and that of the American Medical Association which in 1868 proposed that there be a training school for nurses in every large hospital in the United States.[4]

Thus it is not surprising to read (in the *Concord Monitor*, January 7, 1884) in the seventy-first annual report of the Concord Female Charitable Society the following:

The officers of the Society have found in going about among the poor the great need of some place where the sick poor could have proper care. It is not that they are wanting in affection for each other, always, or that they do not do as well as their circumstances will permit, but the advantage to be gained by the care of trained nurses, the regular attendance of skilled physicians, the comfortable rooms and nourishing food which they do not and cannot have at home, must be apparent to all. We hope that the day is not too far distant when Concord will number among its other notable charities a Hospital, where all who need its shelter can be admitted.

The statistical portion of the report listed aid to fifty-five families: wood, twenty-two cords; two and a half tons of coal; sixty-eight yards of cotton cloth, sixty-seven yards of flannel; food; bedding; and in some cases a nurse. It seems fair to conclude that this report was foremost in the minds of the men and women who gathered to incorporate The Hospital Association on July 3, 1884.

James Lyford's *History of Concord*, which was published in 1903, identifies for us the spark that ignited the flame:

*To the zeal and energy of Dr. Shadrach C. Morrill is due the establish-
ment of the first hospital of Concord which was the first general hospital
of the state. He went among his friends and secured pledges of money before active steps were taken to organize the hospital organization, and when
the nucleus of a sufficient sum had been promised, the first meeting was
called of citizens interested in the subject.*[5]

The following associates organized the hospital under the general laws
of New Hampshire: Shadrach C. Morrill, Samuel C. Eastman, Granville P.
Conn, Parsons B. Cogswell, Charles R. Walker, John A. White, Franklin Low,
Francis L. Abbot, Mrs. Mary Stearns, Henry Bedinger, George Cook, Oliver
Pillsbury, Joseph C.A. Hill, Julia Wallace-Russell, Waldo A. Russell, William Abbott, Rufus P. Staniels, Jesse P. Bancroft, Joseph B. Walker, Henry
J. Crippen. They were the city's leading citizens, bankers, businessmen, physicians, and lawyers. Parsons Cogswell, the editor of the *Concord Monitor*,
later served as mayor. Mary Stevens was the wife of Onslow Stevens, then
superintendent of the Northern Railroad, earlier, governor of New Hampshire. Julia Wallace-Russell was a highly regarded physician whose influence
would prove important to the Concord community within a very few years.

Perhaps it was a hot summer with the cool air of the White Mountains
beckoning, or there may have been differences of opinion on organizational matters, in any case the Hospital Association had many trustees in its earliest days. There were countless resignations and reappointments before the
group settled into the task of leasing a building and making the numerous
decisions attendant upon the task of establishing a hospital. Oliver Pillsbury became the board's first president, a position he occupied for four years.
Francis L. Abbot, who was one of the earliest graduates of St. Paul's School
and associated as secretary with his family's business, Abbot-Downing
Coach Company, served as clerk for the first eleven years of the hospital's
incorporation.

The Bowers house at the corner of Allison and Turnpike streets, called
by many "the balloon house," presumably because of the strange protuber-
ance at the central point of its roof, was leased for two years with an option to buy during that period for $6,000. To orient today's residents of Con-
cord, Turnpike Street was the old name for Route 3, the major route to
Manchester before the completion of Interstate 93. On October 20 the hospital opened and by January 27, 1885, had admitted nine patients, four of
whom were surgical cases. They were cared for by one nurse who, with a
matron and a domestic, constituted the only permanent staff of the new in-

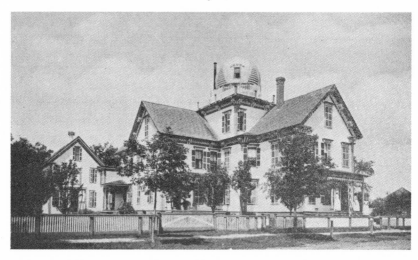

The so-called balloon house at Allison and Turnpike Streets which in October, 1884 became the first unit of the newly incorporated Hospital Association.

stitution. At the end of 1885 four wards had been furnished and occupied.

Six physicians visited the hospital on a rotating basis; Granville Conn, Moses Russell, Ferdinand Stillings, Charles R. Walker, Shadrach Morrill, and Albert Crosby. Eleven additional physicians composed a staff of assistants and consultants for a rapidly increasing patient load. It is not difficult to conclude that the quality of this early medical staff was reassuring to the public for within a few years some twenty towns were represented on the consulting staff, Concord being their nearest medical facility. Clearly the reluctance on the part of the public to use a hospital was quickly fading here. Lilian Carpenter Streeter, an influential Concord citizen and later a trustee of the hospital, was herself a patient during the hospital's second year of existence.[6]

The hospital, as other charitable ventures, became a community effort as can be seen by the list of donations during that first year. John Lamprey furnished the institution with vegetables while Edward Knee made weekly visits to cut hair and shave indigent patients.[7] The city supported two free beds during the first year at a cost of $900. An enterprising trustee, Frances Stevens, suggested the support of a free bed for children to be financed with collections taken in Sunday schools and the gifts of children on occasions such as birthdays. The first year's $50 grew to over $3,000 by 1903 under her stewardship.

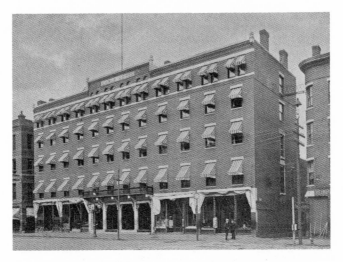

The Eagle Hotel opposite the State House as it appeared in 1899. Later a nursing home, it is now connected to the building at its right anchoring Eagle Market Square.

In October 1885 the donation process was formalized with the establishment of Donation Day, an annual event when volunteers solicited gifts of money, clothing, household articles, and provisions. Not unique to Concord, Donation Day was a fund-raising event employed by most of the early New England voluntary hospitals, surviving well into the mid-twentieth century.

An elaborate set of rules and regulations, developed during the early days of the hospital, governed the actions of trustees, physicians, matron, nurses, even patients. It is evident that abuse of the available free beds was in the minds of trustees who hastened to define carefully the kinds of illness that would be cared for and how such determinations would be made. Patients who paid less than $2 per day were deemed beneficiaries. This figure, incorporated into the hospital's by-laws, had to be periodically altered as the cost of hospitalization rose over the years.

While the trustees established policies and appointed themselves general overseers in the role of the rotating visiting committee, the heaviest load remained for the matron to bear. Mrs. E.A. Sanborn, the first holder of the title, was engaged for the salary of $250 annually to take "general charge of the hospital," a term that encompassed everything from the employment of nurses, purchase of daily supplies, and collection of bills, to the superin-

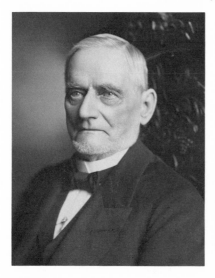 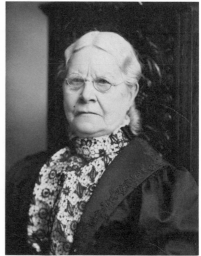

George Alfred Pillsbury, who in dedicating his gift to the city said, "I have been in every state of the union . . . I can truthfully say that if I were to change my present place of residence I know of no city that I should prefer, all things considered, to this city of Concord."

Margaret Sprague Pillsbury, in whose honor the hospital was named "as a token of the love and esteem to the partner of my life, who has for more than fifty years been a true and faithful companion, and has ever shared with me the trials, perplexities and anxieties, as well as the pleasures of these fifty years."

tendence of funeral arrangements of the deceased, including delivery of the body to the family or friends, "obtaining a receipt therefrom."

Nurses (remember, there was only one at first) had merely to care for the patients under the direction of the matron, subject to the physicians' orders. They were directed to "write the directions of the physicians in a daybook provided therefor unless the same is done by the physician."

Realizing the limitations of their small hospital, trustees determined during that first year that they would try to care for acutely ill patients only, those who had some chance of recovery. Rules and regulations stated that if a patient failed to recover after a reasonable time he or she would be discharged. A little later they decided not to admit cases of phthisis, the early name for tuberculosis, endemic among the poor then. In 1886 the trustees voted to decline all lying-in cases, an action which would have far-reaching consequences during the next decade.

Despite the seeming exclusiveness of its clientele, the hospital grew alarmingly and the trustees soon faced the need for expansion. They purchased

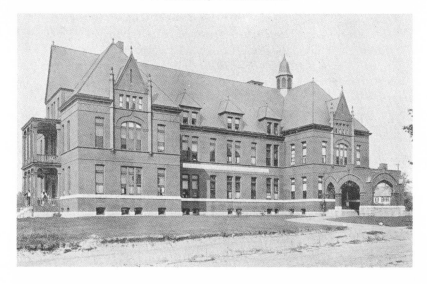

An early view of the Margaret Pillsbury General Hospital. South Main Street was as yet unpaved.

the Bowers house in 1886 with a personal note, appeals to the public having gone unanswered. By 1890 they were $12,000 in debt.

Enter George A. Pillsbury of Minneapolis. On a visit to the state of his
birth, the successful member of the Pillsbury flour milling family was lavish-
ing gifts upon the scenes of his youth — a monument to Civil War dead to
Sutton, a public library to Warner, and on to Concord where he cast about
for a worthy cause. By chance he spoke to John M. Hill who had become
interested in the hospital through a patient of Dr. Ferdinand Stillings. Hill's
statement of Concord's needs led to a correspondence with Dr. Granville
Conn; after working out the details with the physician, an announcement
was made.[8]

George Pillsbury would provide Concord with a hospital. He selected the
site on South Main Street, commissioned the architect, Warren B. Dunnell
of Minneapolis, and supervised construction of the building which cost nearly double his intended gift of $30,000. Ground was broken in September
1890, the dedication presided over by trustee president Samuel Eastman on
October 5, 1891, and the doors opened on December 15.

The profound gratitude (and presumably, relief) of the trustees was expressed through their wish to name the new hospital for Margaret Sprague
Pillsbury, wife of its donor, honoring the Pillsbury's fiftieth wedding an-

niversary. Appropriate toasts were made at an elaborate evening reception at Main Street's Eagle Hotel where Concord citizens mingled with Governor Tuttle, the Pillsburys, city officials, and trustees.[9]

The new hospital was grand indeed with beds for fifty patients, a contagious ward having its own entrance, a classroom for student nurses, and what the trustees deemed plenty of space in the attic for future expansion. It had taken just seven years for the Margaret Pillsbury Hospital to become indispensable to the Concord community.

3

Training Nurses

---

he researcher is unable to find in the most careful reading of the Hospital Association's minutes any formality surrounding the establishment of its training school for nurses. Its existence is mentioned in a matter of fact way early in the first volume, but it is again the *Concord Monitor* which reports on February 1, 1890, that "The course of instruction in the training school for nurses which was established in November has been extended from one and a half to two years." It continues, "Persons who complete the course will be required to pass an examination and will then be given certificates."

The best guess for this apparently casual beginning for the school is that there were few decisions to be made and surely no financial outlay. Pupil nurses became the hospital staff. In fact, starting a training school was the only way to secure a nursing staff. Faculty comprised the superintendent of nurses and those physicians who, having been appointed to the hospital staff, took their turns in three-month blocks visiting the hospital daily to supervise the care of inmates.

Training was rudimentary: a series of lectures by the physicians whose rotations brought them to the hospital, and instruction in the elements of patient care by Miss Mary Barr who was both head nurse and matron at that time. She apparently had her hands full with this double role in which trustees, doctors, pupil-nurses, and patients must be satisfied, and after three years of struggle she left for Manchester's Elliot Hospital.[1]

The Hospital Association Training School for Nurses, as it was then

17

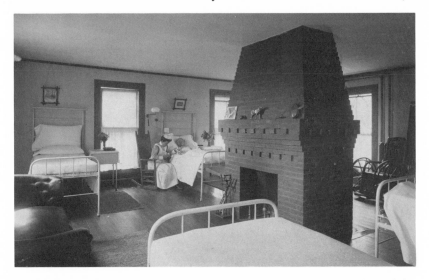

A student nurse takes her patient's pulse in a top floor ward at Pillsbury. Note the gas lights and electric call bell. The hospital was both piped for gas and electrically wired at its construction.

known, required a common school education, that is, an eighth-grade education, and that the prospective pupil possess the scout-like virtues of honesty, sobriety, trustworthiness, and patience, all requisite of well-bred young women of the period. Though little remains to illuminate the daily existence of these women, we know that students were on duty from 7:00 A.M. until 8:00 P.M. with one hour off each day, one afternoon a week and four hours on Sunday. They slept in what became the Stillings ward adjacent to a patient ward to be near their charges. Lectures were held in the evenings and, according to an early account, "If the teacher succeeded in keeping the student awake the lecture was considered a success."

There are a couple of questions research fails to answer concerning the early days of the training school. If the length of the course became two years in February 1890, as the *Monitor* tells us, why do we find three graduates listed for the year 1890? Presumably the first pupils would have completed the course in 1891. It is a mystery too, how pupil nurses could have attended the evening lectures while doing private duty nursing in the city, as we are told they began to do in February 1890.[2] The superintendent of nurses was requested by the trustees to keep a registry of nurses, charging the nurse a fee of 50 cents for each home to which she was sent. Attendance at lectures must have been limited to those pupils who were between assignments

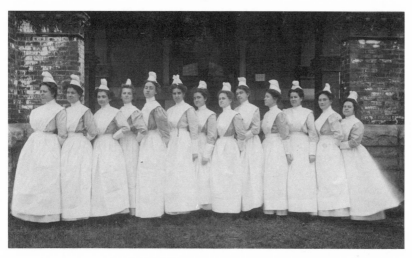

Margaret Pillsbury student nurses pose at the porte cochere of the hospital after the turn of the century. Their starched aprons and cuffs could be changed when soiled, the striped gingham dresses would remain clean. A few of the students have a dark stripe at cap border signifying their advanced status.

or serving their probationary time, a two-month trial during which only the mundane tasks of linen folding, bedmaking, and scrubbing were undertaken. Probationers, who were received at any time of the year, were required to bring with them "three gingham or calico dresses made plainly, three colored washable skirts, eight large white aprons made of bleached cotton, two bags for soiled clothes, one pair of scissors, a napkin ring, a good supply of plain underclothing, every article to be distinctly marked with the owner's name. Nurses are required to wear sensible, well-fitting boots, with rubber heels." Concerning the matter of uniforms, the application stated that upon acceptance into the school the pupil would wear the school uniform. Although we have numerous photographs of students in what appears to be the standard high-necked gingham dress covered by a voluminous white apron worn by students since the late 1870s, there is no documentation of its design. Probably uniforms were made by a local dressmaker according to a pattern chosen by the school.

The newspaper announced one day in March 1890 that Dr. Stillings would lecture to the nurses that month on surgical dressings, poultices, washes, fomentations, bandaging and splints while the following month's lectures by Dr. Chesley would be devoted to circulation, pulse, temperature, respiration, and the secretory and excretory systems including dropsies.[3]

Of the earliest graduates little is known except that one of them, it is believed, was Mary Stillings, daughter of Dr. Ferdinand Stillings, a founder of the hospital and a prominent physician in Concord. It would be interesting to know whether she was encouraged to attend the school to instill confidence in the course of training or whether she was aware that such training could become a valuable asset to her life. It is probable that she served as her father's office nurse in what we presume was a home-office. Sometime prior to 1918 she married a man named Perkins and moved to Jefferson. It is doubtful that she practiced her profession after that time. The practice of nursing, or any other profession, was not deemed suitable for married women then.

The hospital's annual report, a thirty-two-page pamphlet published in March 1890, devoted two pages to the new training school. During the year the duties of head nurse and matron were divided and Miss Harriet Sutherland became head nurse. Miss Sarah Tupper was appointed matron. The report lauded the training school as a most desirable addition to the hospital, its needs identified as better rooms for nurses (this being the year prior to the opening of the new Margaret Pillsbury building) and a ward for contagious cases.[4]

Of the 151 patients treated that year, 27 were outpatients, 11 died. Considering that these represented the poor, that many had sustained serious injuries in railroad accidents or had contaminated wounds from farm mishaps, and that surgery was not lightly undertaken, the number of deaths appears low.

Shortly after the opening of the new hospital — we cannot name the date — it became the site of the first abdominal operation performed under "perfect aseptic detail" in New Hampshire.[5] Dr. Ferdinand Stillings had spent a winter in Philadelphia studying the "details of aseptic surgical work." He brought back with him the necessary materials and supervised drills among the nurses until he was satisfied that they understood this new technique. It was relatively early in the history of asepsis for the techniques to have penetrated to this small New England hospital, for acceptance of the germ theory among American physicians was slow. Almost fifty years had passed since a Hungarian obstetrician had written *The Aetiology, Concept and Prophylaxis of Childbirth Fever*. Pasteur validated his theories in 1864, officially introducing the germ theory to the scientific community. He demonstrated that bacteria could be destroyed by heat and chemical action: pasteurization, of course. After 1865 Joseph Lister developed a method of spraying carbolic acid throughout the operating area and into the wound. His technique further reduced mortality from infection, but it needed refinement since the strong antiseptics used then were often more toxic than the bacteria they killed. As late as 1886 a Philadelphia physician had denounced the germ theory in a sixteen-page paper published in *The Therapeutic Gazette*, but fortunately the realities of reduced mortality due to infection and the constantly improving aseptic techniques began to convince physicians of the need for absolute cleanliness. By the turn of the century aseptic surgery had become universally accepted.[6]

Anesthesia was in use as well and, with the 1895 discovery of the x-ray and the advent of blood transfusion, the hospital became the preferred site for surgery. It was far easier to prepare the newly developed operating room for a surgical procedure than to create aseptic conditions in the patient's home no matter how palatial that dwelling might be.

Two emergency situations tested the Pillsbury staff shortly before the turn of the century. The first, a wreck of the White Mountain Express at Ferry Street, Concord, in 1896, caused the death of two and injured eighteen. All were treated at the Margaret Pillsbury Hospital with help from Manchester's Elliot Hospital and from Boston. Two years later a sudden demand for care occurred when soldiers of the First Regiment of Volunteers were sent home from field hospitals during the Spanish American War. Sixty-four cases of typhoid fever and a few malaria victims received hospital care. Only four typhoid patients died though many were in very poor condition upon their arrival in Concord.[7]

When the twentieth century dawned it found Concord with two general hospitals, a state institution for mental illness, and three training schools for nurses.

4

A Hospital for Women

ulia Eastman Wallace graduated from the Women's Medical College of the New York Infirmary in 1877. A year later, after serving an internship in Boston's New England Hospital for Women and Children, she arrived in Concord to establish a medical practice. She and Dr. Mary Danforth of Manchester became the first women admitted to the New Hampshire Medical Society (1878).

A native of Hill, New Hampshire, Dr. Wallace quickly built a large practice statewide in scope. An article written about Julia by her sister Ellen, also a physician, for the *Medical Woman's Journal* mentions that before her marriage to Waldo Russell in 1882, she regularly took patients into her home for care.[1] When this was no longer possible (Did her husband object?) she began to worry about these out-of-town patients who needed care, particularly those who could not afford a private hospital room. Remembering that the Margaret Pillsbury Hospital did not admit lying-in cases and that indigent patients were, as beneficiaries, seen by the physician on service, it is unlikely that these poor women could be treated by a woman physician at all. Not one was on the active attending staff of any hospital in New Hampshire.

It is surely an injustice typical of the period that, although Dr. Wallace-Russell had been an incorporator of the Pillsbury institution, lecturing to the earliest pupils in its training school, she was barred from caring for her own patients in the hospital unless they were able to pay the full cost of private care there.

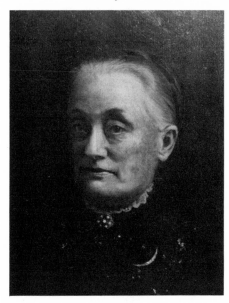

Julia Wallace-Russell, a founder of the New Hamp-
shire Memorial Hospital for Women and Children,
from a portrait by Caroline Savery Kenyon. She
and her husband Waldo Russell were also incorpor-
ators of the original Hospital Association.

On September 12, 1895, a few women gathered with Dr. Wallace-Russell in her 44 Pleasant Street home to form the Women's Hospital Aid Association. They were: Mrs. Louise F. Richards, Newport, Mary Ann Downing, Concord, Mrs. Caroline R. Thyng, Laconia, and Dr. Ellen Wallace, Manchester. A surviving copy of the organization's constitution states:

The objects of this Association shall be: First- To raise funds in any proper way for the purpose of aiding poor women and children of the State of New Hampshire in times of sickness that wish to be under the care of women physicians. Second- To provide such places for them either in hospitals or private homes, as the times and circumstances demand, or in any way authorized by the trustees. Third- To hold in trust "The Julia Wallace-Russell Fund" or any other funds that may be legally entrusted or bequeathed to said association. And primarily we would make these funds a fitting monument to women's medical work, and leave it as a token of love to those who shall come after us, for their mutual care and munificence.[2]

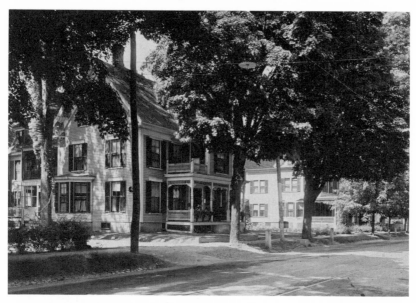

Only a small sign at the right of the front door identified this house at 66 South Street as the New Hampshire Hospital for Women and Children in the early years of the twentieth century.

The fund had been designed and monies solicited to pay the hospital expenses for indigent women so that they might be treated by their women physicians, but the idea of a women's hospital grew rapidly. Mrs. Vasta Abbott of 66 South Street, who planned to leave the house to the organization, died unexpectedly before she could do so. Her brother, heir to the house, also died soon after so that the organization was able to purchase it for $7,000 in the fall of 1896. On October 10 the first patient was admitted to what must have been a hastily fitted up New Hampshire Memorial Hospital for Women and Children. Operating income was derived from contributions, bequests, and memberships. A $100 donor became a patron; $25 entitled one to a life membership, and $1 annually allowed the giver a vote at association meetings.[3]

Within a year (October 1, 1897) a training school was in operation under the supervision of Esther Dart. Much like its neighboring institution, students heard lectures from visiting physicians, and by 1903 eleven women had graduated from the two-year course.

It was not long after the advent of this competition that the trustees of the Margaret Pillsbury Hospital began to examine some early decisions. In

1900, upon investigation by a committee, lying-in cases were admitted at a cost of $15 per week. About the same time the training school course was lengthened to three years and a case of phthisis was admitted on a private basis as an experiment. Evidently the idea of a supporting organization or auxiliary began to interest the trustees too, for they appointed a committee of the women trustees to explore the formation of what they called a "Ladies Aid Society." Despite the free bed funds money was tight, every jar of jelly contributed on Donation Day gratefully received and acknowledged in the hospital's annual report. The possibility of an organized group of women working actively to raise funds for the hospital must have appeared exceedingly attractive to the trustees although not attractive enough to initiate action; the Margaret Pillsbury Chapter, as they called their auxiliary, was not created until 1926.

While we have been looking at New England, what was happening in the rest of the country? Training schools proliferated greatly around the turn of the century for hospitals could not exist without the patient care students provided, hiring graduate nurses to staff patient wards remained far in the future. In 1880 there were 15 schools, 20 years later the number was 432.[4] Naturally the large prestigious schools such as Bellevue's and that of Johns Hopkins Hospital in Baltimore received large numbers of applicants and were thus able to attract students of the highest calibre. It would become a continuing struggle for the smallest schools to graduate more than a few nurses each year, a struggle that translated to an inadequate staff caring for patients in these hospitals. Too, these small institutions could not offer the number of patients or variety of cases needed to provide a comprehensive education for pupil nurses.

Our two fledgling training schools appear to have been carefully managed during the early years; each turned out a small but steady stream of graduate nurses who went out to do private duty work or served as physicians' office nurses in Concord and throughout the United States and Canada. At one point a private hospital in Franklin asked to be supplied with senior nurses at $10 per month. This was the stipend paid (in 1904) to nurses in training at Margaret Pillsbury. Trustees were careful not to call this small sum a salary, for students' work in the hospital was considered an even exchange for training received. Even though there were frequent epidemics of diphtheria, scarlet fever, and smallpox, the Concord area must have become oversupplied with nurses around 1911. The trustees of the Margaret Pillsbury Hospital voted that year not to accept Concord residents who applied to its training school except by a special vote of the trustees. During this period the New Hampshire Memorial School was graduating about a half-dozen nurses a year and the New Hampshire Hospital School was sending another dozen or so into the community.

Of concern to Margaret Pillsbury's trustees in 1914 was the problem of physicians bringing their office nurses to the hospital to assist in the operating room. Trustees voted to prohibit this custom for all but the senior men of the advisory staff in order that pupil nurses could receive essential training in operative procedures.

Conduct and self-discipline among nurses in training were of great importance to trustees, hospital administrators, and nursing instructors, but of paramount importance to the pupils themselves if they were to successfully conclude their training. All of the old fashioned virtues of self-denial, obedience, and devotion to duty, characteristic of the early religious orders and the military background of the Nightingale model, were considered appropriate to the nursing profession at the turn of the century and for many years beyond. The probationary period varying from two to six months was designed, as was the novitiate, to discover hidden weaknesses of character or undesirable qualities that could render a woman unfit for nursing. Hospital superintendents traded disciplinary methods most of which involved extra hours of duty and more work.

All this discipline caused a great deal of illness among pupil nurses who were expected to be on duty nearly year round with little time for socializing and few vacations. *The Advance of American Nursing* devotes much space to the description of eighty- and ninety- hour work weeks for nurses at a time when the average for industry was around fifty-seven hours. A disproportionate amount of work time was lost to flat and painful feet and to acute digestive disturbances. While today's students lose time to mononucleosis, housemaid's knee was frequently diagnosed at the turn-of-the-century.[5]

In Concord the pattern was similar. Monthly reports of the superintendent of Margaret Pillsbury Hospital attest to the high degree of illness among students who at times required nursing themselves. The attrition rate among probationers was high due to the drudgery demanded of them. Laura Meader, superintendent at the Pillsbury Hospital reported to trustees in April 1917 that, of the two probationers admitted during the month, one had resigned "after being on duty two days, did not like 'cleaning.'" Three applications had been received that were "not satisfactory in any way." She announced to trustees that "beginning next week, we are going to have a short prayer service at 6:35 A.M., lasting about five minutes which will not only start the day right, but will mean that the nurses will all be at breakfast at a more regular time."[6]

Long hours, drudgery unrelated to education, sending students half-educated into private homes to enrich the hospitals' coffers — all this had not continued unnoticed by nursing educators. As early as 1893 when the Columbian Exposition was held in Chicago, it attracted many congresses and conferences, among them an international congress of charities and philanthropic organizations. A section was devoted to hospital care of the sick, the training of nurses and dispensary (outpatient) work and first aid to the injured. Isabel Hampton, superintendent of the Johns Hopkins Hospital Training School, was chairman of a subsection on nursing. She had previously warned that schools which desired to lengthen their training periods to three years would do so at their own peril if they did not also shorten the nurses' work week.

The American Society of Superintendents of Training Schools was founded at this meeting. At its first gathering in 1894 forty-four superintendents attended, creating a movement that would serve as the catalyst for the formation of the first national organization for nurses, the Nurses' Associated Alumnae of the United States and Canada. From this group a committee on periodicals, feeling that a magazine to represent nursing was needed, created the *American Journal of Nursing*, its first issue dated October 1900.[7] Nursing now had an organizational focus and a voice to speak for its interests. Hospitals too were beginning to organize with the advent of the American Hospital Association in 1899.

In Concord trustees of the Margaret Pillsbury Hospital, having survived the rigors of birth and rapid growth, began to decentralize their control of the institution. They established standing committees to oversee its day-to-day operation in the areas of finance, free beds and trust funds, nurses, and buildings and grounds.

5

Social Reform and the Great War

apid change became the norm as the city and its hospitals grew. The pages of Margaret Pillsbury's trustee records were filled with reports of gifts creating free bed funds, instrument funds, additions to the building. The Foster ward for children was constructed and equipped in 1902 using a $3,000 gift in memory of William Lawrence Foster, Harriet Morton Foster, and Roger Elliott Foster. The next year Dr. Stillings' wife furnished the female surgical ward to be known as the Stillings ward. In 1904 the John H. Pearson fund built an addition to the west side of the building consisting of a basement laundry, nurses' and servants' dining rooms on the first floor, and a four-room maternity ward to be designated the Pearson ward on the second floor.[1]

During these years many of the hospital's original staff members passed away: Dr. Shadrach Morrill in 1904, Drs. Frederick Cummings and Andros Chesley in 1908, Ralph Gallinger in 1911 and Granville Conn in 1916. Memorial Hospital lost its founder and physician-in-charge Julia Wallace-Russell in 1906.

Mrs. Abbie Moseley provided a two-story addition to the south side of the Pillsbury building in 1916 in memory of her husband. Each of the two six-bed wards was glassed and screened with awnings creating what were then known as open-air wards, providing a popular treatment for respiratory illnesses such as TB. Patients spent a portion of the day here under heavy blankets absorbing fresh air, thought to have great curative powers. Some hospitals, notably the TB sanatoria of the Adirondacks, placed their beds on tracks enabling them to be wheeled straight out through doors onto open air porches.

Relations between the two hospitals appear to have been cordial. Some physicians served both institutions. The same Mrs. Vasta Abbott whose home became Memorial Hospital provided a $5,000 free bed fund in her will for the Pillsbury Hospital, and on more than one occasion trustees of the two hospitals conferred before establishing rate schedules. In the matter of fund raising, however, Pillsbury's trustees voted not to participate in a common fund drive with Memorial in 1914. Their reasons for this decision and a later decision (1922) not to join with Memorial to form a single hospital are nowhere explained. Even though the recommendation came from the Merrimack County Medical Society the move was "deemed inadvisable."

Pillsbury's training school began to enlarge its scope of activity realizing a need for a greater diversity of patients. In 1912 trustees authorized the superintendent to affiliate with "some children's hospital." Now that there were two hospitals in town both would be competing for the few young patients who were seriously ill or in need of surgery. It appears that the hospital chosen was the Boston Free Dispensary. Two years later the training school became affiliated with the Concord District Nursing Association. This experience would ensure that students saw how the poor lived, teaching them to improvise as they not only tended the sick but instructed families in the elements of sanitation, nutrition, and such disease prevention as was known then.

Although training schools were graduating nurses in many parts of the country, numerous women continued to find employment as nurses without the benefit of any form of training. Some type of registration for nurses was needed to protect the public. South Africa had become the first country to recognize this need, adopting legislation in 1891. Britain followed in 1901, but the democratic government of the United States required that such legislation originate at the state level. Sophia Palmer broached the subject in a paper read before the New York State Federation of Women's Clubs in 1898. The Federation's response was a resolution in favor of a board of examiners to be chosen by the state society of nurses. It was recommended that the Board of Regents of the State University of New York supervise the work of the examiners in regulating nursing. Impetus for immediate action on the matter came in 1900 with the announcement that the Philadelphia County Medical Society and College of Physicians would establish a school of nursing to prepare nurses in only ten weeks. At the same time correspondence schools sprang up, promising that anyone could become a trained nurse in a few months of study at home. The impressive diploma would fool the public and place its owner on the same level as the authentically trained graduate nurse.

The following year the newly formed International Council of Nurses framed a resolution that demanded the states' cooperation in passing legislation regulating the education of nurses and securing state examinations to validate nurse registration. North Carolina's was the first bill to pass amid a flurry of state organizations formed to push registration bills through state legislatures. New York's law was considered the best, requiring that nurses be graduates of training schools approved by regents of the state university. Nurses not trained in New York, who were employed privately or by institutions, were required to register in accordance with the new law to continue work in New York. Schools outside New York hastened to register with the Board of Regents to allow their graduates to work in that state. Some altered teaching methods and broadened curricula to conform to New York State's requirements. One course required by New York State's Board of Nurse Examiners was obstetrics, a subject not being taught by many training schools. Eagerness to conform to the New York requirements brought about the establishment of obstetrics courses in schools throughout the east.[2]

New Hampshire passed its Nurse Practice Act on March 7, 1907, its four provisions creating a rudimentary form of control over the profession.[3] They placed responsibility for carrying out the act with the regent of the State Board of Medical Examiners. A state registration by examination of graduate nurses was established for graduates of schools giving a course of at least two years. A three-year waiver was granted to nurses already in practice as well as students in schools. Registrants paid a fee of five dollars. The final provision called for the appointment of five nurse examiners to serve as inspectors of schools who would be nominated by the New Hampshire Graduate Nurses' Association. These examiners were to be appointed by the aforementioned regent.

This overall supervision of nurse registration was transferred to the Superintendent of Public Institutions in a 1915 amendment. Four years later that office was abolished in favor of a Commissioner of Education acting for a State Board of Education. The waiver clause was omitted when the Nurse Practice Act was rewritten in 1925.

Concomitant with the regulation of nursing were the earliest attempts at control over the way medicine was practiced in the hospital. The 1920 Flexner report to the Carnegie Foundation for the Advancement of Teaching was responsible for major reform in medical education.[4] Abraham Flexner had visited personally every one of the nation's 155 medical schools finding them in the main sadly wanting. His examination of entrance requirements, size

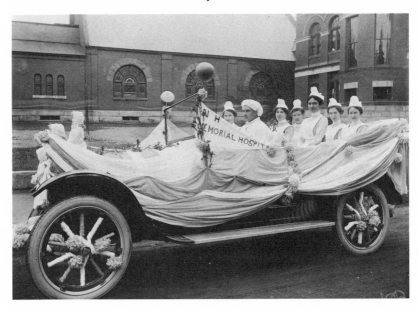

Student nurses from Memorial Hospital and their attired-for-surgery driver in a 1915 parade celebrating Concord's 150th anniversary. They are shown passing Concord High School and the Unitarian Church located in the block now occupied by the New Hampshire Savings Bank.

and quality of faculty, physical facilities, financial support, and relationship to hospitals was reported in detail with no concessions to the sensibilities. Conditions were described as "disgraceful," "shameful," and "foul." Institutions hastened to correct the situation by means of mergers and affiliations with universities, but, predictably, the weaker schools perished. The decade of 1910 to 1920 saw medical education strengthened as a new university discipline.

As for hospitals, shortly after its founding in 1913, the American College of Surgeons took on the regulatory function beginning with study and analytical work aimed at the organization and standardization of management. During 1918 and 1919 hospitals of one hundred beds or more in the United States and Canada were visited by representatives of the college who surveyed ten areas in each institution including the physical plant, organizational structure and governing board, medical staff, diagnostic and therapeutic facilities, medical records, and "humanitarian spirit in which the best care of the patient is always the primary consideration." During the first year 89 hospitals met their standards; the second year the number grew to 198.[5]

Neither Margaret Pillsbury nor Memorial Hospital were large enough to have been visited, but we have evidence from trustee records that at Pillsbury Hospital physicians were well aware of these efforts to improve hospital management. To Dr. Carleton Metcalf belongs the credit for introducing the matter of medical records to trustees in a report dated 1921:

Dr. C.R. Metcalf was present and suggested various changes in the matter of hospital records and additional equipment. Dr. Metcalf advocated a record of each operation dictated to a nurse on completion of operations by the operating surgeon and that a certain nurse be employed to make the records of all cases in permanent form, including brief history of the case on entrance to the hospital, record of the operation, and brief record of subsequent medication.

On June 21, 1921 trustees voted that the history of all cases admitted to the hospital, except those of outpatients, be taken, records to be confidential, except for the requirements of attending and personal physicians. The hospital promised to provide forms for these histories to be completed by the attending physician, except that operative records would be taken by the anesthetist in attendance and approved by the operating surgeon. Records would not be taken from the hospital except by vote of the trustees. Furthermore, a separate motion authorized the superintendent's purchase of suitable desks for the storage of charts and completion of records. Prohibition, now in force, created its own need for records as hospitals were required to execute a bond and apply to the United States Treasury Department to obtain alcohol for medicinal use, and such use had to be justified by report of the superintendent.

By now, World War I, called by many the Great War, had been concluded. Records of trustee meetings from that period convey almost none of the drama being played out here in Concord as well as in training camps and on battlefields across the Atlantic.

One of the best and most moving accounts of the nurse's daily existence at the front in France comes from Vera Brittain, a young Englishwoman who postponed an Oxford education to care for the wounded in French hospitals. *Testament of Youth*, written from the prospective of 1933, eloquently chronicles the horrors she experienced in attempting to nurse British and French soldiers in improvised, inadequate, and overcrowded hospitals after an equally inadequate training in London.[6]

Here in Concord patriotism fairly shone from the pages of the *Concord*

Evening Monitor. Every battle, every advance was cheered in the headlines and first-hand accounts gleaned from letters sent home by the sons of Concord citizens were quoted at length bringing the action closer to home. Concord sent at least nine physicians off to war. Drs. Russell Wilkins, Carleton Metcalf, Henry Amsden, Harold Conner, and Robert Blood went to France, while Drs. Dennis Sullivan, Robert Graves, and Charles Quinn served in training camps in this country. Dr. Marion Bugbee of Memorial Hospital spent six months in France. Her experiences there were the subject of a talk given to the Associates, the volunteer organization at Memorial, on her return.

Pillsbury's training school supplied seventeen graduates to war service. Josephine Barrett of the class of 1914 died at Camp Greenleaf, Georgia, while serving in the Red Cross. Adruenna Allen Tupper who graduated in 1894 died in Uxbridge, England, in December 1916. She had been decorated with the Royal Red Cross by King George at Buckingham Palace for extraordinary service at Salisbury Plain and in France. She was buried with full military honors at Uxbridge.[7]

The joy felt by those at home upon the conclusion of the war in the late fall of 1918 was tempered by the great loss of lives suffered in the worldwide influenza epidemic. Spread by returning soldiers the disease began gradually in September reaching a devastating peak by November.

It had been a busy summer in the city. The end of the war was in sight with encouraging progress in the Allied advancement in France. Long lists of the names of men of draft age filled the paper and one imagines a great deal of anxious talk among residents who saw the draft numbers next to the names of sons, friends, and relatives. The usual summer outings and picnics must have been attended largely by the very young and elderly since there were few men between the ages of eighteen and forty-five available. Indeed, women were busy as well, holding jobs formerly done by men, knitting for the soldiers, nursing.

Major league baseball was still in the news at the beginning of the season. The *Monitor* reported on July 10 that "the baseball sensation of this season is 'Babe Ruth' of the Boston Americans." A week later the word was "The big league teams are losing their stars very rapidly as the men enlist in military or naval service, respond to the draft or leave the diamond to engage in 'useful employments.'"

The first report of influenza carried by the *Monitor* told of 65 deaths at Camp Devens (now Fort Devens) in 24 hours with 5-6,000 cases under treatment there. By September 25 Concord had 80 cases, Manchester 600. Residents were urged to remain at home if ill. A day later 102 cases were report-

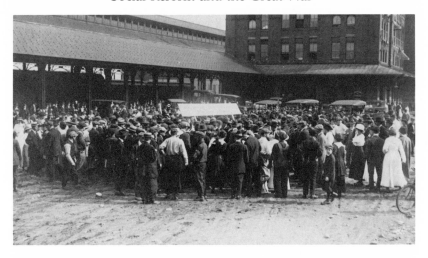

On what appears to be a warm September 20, 1917, families and friends crowded the yard at the railroad station to see off Concord's young enlistees in World War I. Their sign held aloft reads: "We're from the Capital of New Hampshire to the Capital of Germany."

ed, the day after that 204. Churches closed. By the 30th schools and theatres closed. People who had taken Red Cross courses in first aid and home nursing were asked to volunteer to care for families in Concord. It was not unusual for entire families to be ill at the same time rendering them helpless. Those who owned automobiles were requested to volunteer them to speed district nurses on their rounds. Dr. Chancy Adams describes the involvement of the city's hospitals:

In 1918 the Hospital [Pillsbury], as all hospitals in the State again stood the acid test when the city was filled with those sick and dying from influenza, an epidemic unprecedented in the history of the State and Nation. Of the 26 nurses in our hospital 25 were ill. This calamity, together with the absence of eight of our physicians in the Service, proved a great handicap to the efficiency of the Hospital. It was necessary to establish an emergency hospital as the burden of sickness became too heavy for the two hospitals to carry. The Elk's Home was opened for that purpose and functioned until the crisis was over. What an experience. For a time it was impossible to obtain caskets enough to care for the dead.[8]

On October 5 the city board of health recommended that "only kinsmen and very near friends attend the last rites of people who die during this period." It was decided that men students at New Hampshire College (the name for the state university in Durham) would sleep in tents adopting the War Department regulations to safeguard the health of students. Women students were asked not to report to school until notified so that the incubation period of the men might pass before introducing a new group to the college environment.

A feeling of anticipation was in the air despite the gravity of the epidemic. Advertisements for flags competed with those of undertakers for space between the headlines. On Tuesday, October 24, came the announcement that epidemic regulations against gatherings and community events would be lifted the following Saturday at midnight.

Concord was ready for the celebration which erupted in the streets as the Associated Press flashed the news to the *Monitor* moments after the armistice was proclaimed. Bells rang from the Central Fire Station and the North End tower. Local officials had arranged to detonate twenty-five aerial bombs to signal acceptance of the terms offered Germany by Marshall Foch. Feeling that a formal celebration was in order, the city planned to hold a parade on Main Street the following Monday.

FIREWORKS   BAND   BONFIRE
All the fixings Come One Come All

You will never celebrate like this again for a better cause. Don't leave the noise at home.[9]

6

People and Progress

ursing was at a low ebb at the conclusion of the war. Many nurses had perished abroad and many more were lost to the influenza epidemic. Some were unable to continue in the profession due to the lasting effects of the illness. Now that the glamour of serving one's country had diminished, the large number of women who had entered nursing schools in a fever of patriotism was greatly reduced. Students left without finishing their training and hospitals were unable to care for patients as well as their increasingly improving standards now required.

During the war and epidemic the spotlight had focused on nurses because of the great public dependence on them. For the first time it became evident that the training furnished nurses was vastly inadequate. Furthermore, there was only one collegiate program training nurse educators, the one begun at Columbia Teacher's College in 1914. Margaret Pillsbury Hospital was fortunate to recognize the need for and hire a Teacher's College educator, Mary C. Gilmore, also an alumna of the Peter Bent Brigham Hospital School, who came in 1920, the first nurse in Concord to devote all her time to teaching. According to an account in the annual report for 1934 which chronicled the history of the school, she had a minimum amount of classroom equipment, teaching in a frame house on Main Street south of the hospital building. Osma Morrill, widow of founder Shadrach Morrill was then chairman of the committee on nurses. As a member of the city department of education she was keenly interested in the school and responsible for many improvements made in the course of study during the twenties. Incidentally, it was

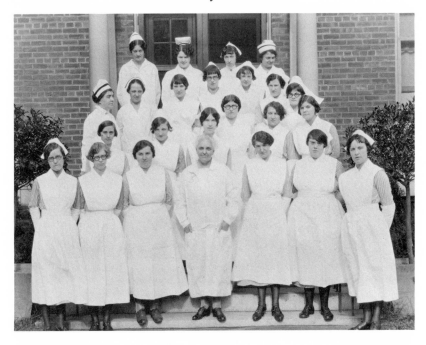

Memorial Hospital's nursing school class of 1927 with their instructors and Dr. Marion Bugbee.

at the suggestion of Mrs. Morrill that the Margaret Pillsbury Chapter was formed in 1926. The work of the auxiliary augmented the hospital's financial resources while adding many pleasant extras to the hospital visits of patients and the nurses' training school years.

During the twenties and thirties a recurrent theme of annual reports to the trustees from the superintendent of the hospital was the need for a department of nursing within the state university to enable promising graduates to further their training. These nurses would be equipped to provide better clinical training to students who could then provide better bedside nursing. Although there were twenty-five colleges and universities with nursing programs leading to the A.B. or B.S. degree by the mid-twenties, only one of them, Simmons College, was located in New England. Even so, Alma Van Pelt, superintendent of nurses in 1934, proudly detailed the postgraduate plans of three of her recent students, hinting broadly that a scholarship in support of postgraduate education immediately following graduation from the School of Nursing would, as she put it, "stimulate endeavor among the students and make possible a closer correlation between the Nursing School and institutions of higher learning."[1]

The last five years of the twenties were devoted to planning, raising money for, and erecting a nurses' residence to serve the Pillsbury Hospital. Graduate nurses who held positions of authority and students in training, the hospital's nursing staff, shared these new quarters, a businesslike brick building adjacent to the hospital, today occupied by McKerley's Nursing Home. The Blue Cross-Blue Shield building across the street occupies the site of the original "balloon house."

Harry G. Emmons, owner of the Main Street department store bearing his name was in general charge of the drive to raise $250,000. With such division leaders as Frank J. Sulloway and James M. Langley, the amount realized was over $335,000. The young Langley, publisher and editor of the *Concord Monitor* beginning in 1923, was cutting his fund-raising teeth on this project and learning about the hospital business. He would be heard from again.

During the twenties which may have roared elsewhere, sober Concord citizens were toiling to enlarge the Memorial Hospital, too. Dr. Marion Bugbee, who became physician-in-charge at the death of Julia Wallace-Russell, worked to increase the hospital's services. With the help of Dr. Carleton Metcalf she established an orthopedic clinic to serve children from throughout the state. When a fund drive to raise $100,000 was announced in 1921, headed by local jeweler J.C. Derby, the addition to be built with its proceeds was described as space for maternity wards, an orthopedic operating room, plaster rooms, and a small gymnasium for children. To have a capacity of twenty-five beds, it would make space available elsewhere in the building for twelve additional medical and surgical patients.

Hospitals were becoming more popular for childbirth. More sophisticated obstetrical care demanded anesthesia for birth and thus the scrubbed atmosphere of the delivery room. Dr. Bugbee explained that "nearly all first babies are born in hospitals now because the majority of young couples are not suitably situated in their own homes for the event." She added, "Women who have several children prefer hospital care," their one chance for a rest. In that year, one-third of the 419 births in Concord took place at Memorial Hospital.[2]

There was some criticism expressed by potential donors who had heard that outside fund raisers were to run the drive, that $10,000 would be siphoned off from funds collected by local volunteers. Chairman Derby hastened to correct this impression explaining that funds had been given es-

pecially to pay the fund raisers and every penny collected would go directly to the hospital enlargement. He promised an itemized statement of gifts
and expenses (if any) of the campaign.

The addition designed by George Griffin of Concord was a project of the
thirteen-year-old Hospital Associates, the women's auxiliary. The women,
who had added to their treasury, bazaar by bazaar, until they had accumu-
lated the purchase price of the Spring Street lot adjoining the rear of the main
building. At the Associates' October 1921 annual meeting the building fund
and coming public campaign were the chief topics of discussion. Speakers
extolled the quality of care offered by the hospital, claiming that the highest
rate for a private room was less than the cost of a private nurse at home.
They emphasized the care given elderly women in their last illnesses and
those suffering from chronic and incurable ailments. A number of elderly
women of means had even made the hospital their home in their declining
years, a service not offered by any other hospital in the state.

Thirty teams of women and ten of men, numbering 330, fanned out across
Concord and surrounding towns, their progress marked by a large
electrically-lighted clock on the building north of the Masonic Temple. Boy
Scout troops No. 1 and No. 6 of the YMCA distributed window cards to
be displayed by stores and factories. Among those receiving an early ex-
posure to eleemosynary activity were Arthur Virgin, Haven Huckins, Dudley Orr, Kingsley Batchelder, Holbrook Horton, Edward Amsden, George
Witham, and Edson Phelps. One of the more dubious forms of publicity
indulged in by the enthusiastic fund raisers was the window display at Main
Street's David E. Murphy Store. It was a live presentation of children in various states of orthopedic repair accompanied by two nurses. Advertisements
for the drive appeared in the newspapers portraying these unfortunate victims of congenital malformations, accidents, and malnutrition. This form
of appeal to the public probably presaged the poster child of the fifties and
later who aided drives for polio and muscular dystrophy.

That month (September) the newspapers described a "brilliant reception"
concluding the Memorial Hospital's training school graduation exercises.
Among those present to congratulate graduates were Dr. Bugbee, Dr. and
Mrs. Loren Sanders, Dr. Robert O. Blood, Harriet Huntress of the New
Hampshire Education Department, nurses from the Margaret Pillsbury
Hospital and Concord's district nurses Clara Mitchell, Florence Morrill, and
Anne Allen. The reception's honoree was Mrs. Alfred Melanson of Wey-
mouth, Nova Scotia, whose five daughters had all come to Concord to train
as nurses. Two had already graduated from Memorial's school, two were
in training there, and one was a Margaret Pillsbury graduate.

The campaign was heralded daily in Concord's two newspapers. Even the *Union Leader* in neighboring Manchester contributed an editorial in praise of this laudable effort. Teams of men and women returned from their visits with stories of personal sacrifice. Every contribution was acknowledged in the papers. Concord's three motion picture theatres contributed the proceeds of a Wednesday evening performance in addition to the display of slides and the presentation of four-minute speeches by campaign chairman J.C. Derby, men's division chairman, Olin Chase, and Judge James Remick.

Workers who attended the weekly report meetings, more in the nature of pep rallies, were fed by the Girl Scouts, ladies aid societies and, on the last official day of the drive, by the ladies of the Swedish Society. On that October 28, 1921, only $74, 599 was reported. Workers were exhorted to bring in additional subscriptions until the $100,000 was achieved. Presumably the campaign reached its goal eventually, for the next clipping in Associates President Mrs. W.F. Nelson's scrapbook, reports on the cornerstone-laying ceremony the following December with Dr. Ellen Wallace, last surviving founder of the hospital, presiding. The tin box cemented into the cornerstone of the new maternity ward contained early records of the hospital, pictures of founders Julia Wallace-Russell and Mary Ann Downing, the bylaws of the Associates, campaign folders and press notices concerning the recent drive, and a piece of money for good luck.

On June 30, 1924, the wing was dedicated with splendid ceremony. It was noted in one newspaper account that the words "New Hampshire Memorial Hospital" over the entrance were carved by Joseph J. Comi of Concord. Despite the building's years of use by others, those words are in evidence today on South Spring Street.

The name Winant figures heavily in the annals of both hospitals during this period. Son of a wealthy New York family, John Gilbert Winant was born in 1889.[3] He attended St. Paul's School and Princeton, returning to St. Paul's after service in World War I to teach history. Captivated by politics, he rose rapidly through the General Court to the Senate, then served three terms as governor. During these years he was a trustee of the Margaret Pillsbury Hospital, chairing the training school committee and giving generously to the work of the hospital. At the time of the Memorial fund drive his gift of $2,000 was one of the largest individual contributions received. During the Depression when the Memorial Hospital was struggling to meet financial obligations, Governor Winant offered to reduce the price of the milk he furnished the hospital from his farm, a gesture gratefully received by trustees.

Of the several governors of New Hampshire who have been associated with Concord's hospitals, John Winant's life of selfless service, international in scope, is a model for any age. His career took him from the State House in Concord to Washington where he helped draft the Social Security Act, then served on the Social Security Board. He resigned as Republican minority member of the board to support Franklin Roosevelt's second presidential campaign when Republican candidate Alf Landon repudiated the Social Security Act. Winant returned to the board for two months to finish the task of registering the first old-age pensioners. Believing that the United States' membership in the International Labor Organization was a way to hold some influence over events he felt were moving toward war, Winant returned to direct that organization with which he had worked earlier. In January 1941 President Roosevelt appointed him Ambassador to Great Britain. He was with Winston Churchill at 10 Downing Street on the evening the radio news announced the Japanese bombing of Pearl Harbor, an evening he remembers in his memoir of those momentous times, *Letter from Grovesnor Square*. Winant served as ambassador until 1946, dying in 1947. His gravestone in St. Paul's School cemetery bears an exerpt from his writings which includes the words " . . . without charity there can be no good."

A little later the lure of politics brought physician Robert O. Blood to New Hampshire's highest office. Like Winant, Blood, an Enfield native and Dartmouth Medical School graduate, had come to the capital city as a young man. He established a practice as a physician and surgeon, and was appointed to the Margaret Pillsbury staff in 1916. He too entered World War I, as a first lieutenant in the medical corps. When he returned to Concord he was a major, having earned, among other decorations, the Croix de Guerre of France. During his more than fifty years of active practice in Concord he was also a businessman, the owner of a dairy, and a farmer, the owner and operator of Crystal Springs Farm, where he bred prize-winning Ayreshire cattle. He became a legislator, moving from the House to the Senate of which he was president in 1939. His two terms as governor were followed by years of dedication to the Republican party including attendance as a delegate at three Republican national conventions.[4]

Although a study in contrasts personally, the two men had much in common including their interest in and work on behalf of Pillsbury, Memorial, and Concord hospitals.

The Depression was particularly hard on Memorial Hospital. Smaller than Pillsbury it served a narrower range of patients, and after the advent of the orthopedic clinic, fewer paying patients. These children were often poor and confined to the hospital for long periods of time. It is difficult to tell from the records available whether the hospital was actually mis-

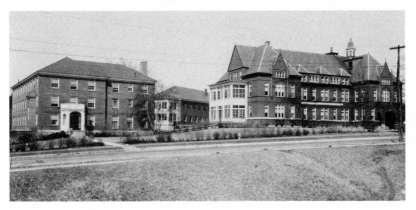

Kimball Studio took this view of the Pillsbury Hospital for the 1934 annual report. The building to the left of the now glassed-in porches was the nurses' residence. The annex, later the Concord Clinic, is between the two buildings.

managed; we do know that collection of bills was slow. A few patients who owed the hospital asked to work out their debts in their trades. Mattresses were made over at two dollars each, pillows were made from a donated feather bed. Furniture bequeathed to the hospital thriftily augmented or replaced worn out items.

The trustees reluctantly concluded that the old wooden structure on South Street should be closed, and they arranged to make a few renovations to the new brick building to house all patients. It would be cheaper to heat and require less maid service.

The training school had been doing well. Three students were studying at Yale University's nursing program, an affiliation arranged with the well-known nursing educator Annie Goodrich, its superintendent at the time. It lasted only one year, though. Yale was oversupplied with affiliations and Memorial's, the most recent, was the first to be terminated. Despite its success trustees were determined to explore every opportunity to save money so they discussed closing the school in favor of an all-graduate nursing staff. This idea was discarded as too expensive and trustees decided to pay students a sliding scale of monthly stipends: $5 to first year students, $6 for the second year, and $7 for the third year. A total of $1608 was saved over the flat rate payment of $10.50 to all. They agreed upon a 5 percent reduction in staff salaries.

The medical staff was understandably unhappy about the consolidation of patients into the South Street building. It would be crowded, noisy, and inconvenient for patients and staff. The move was accomplished amid rumblings of dissatisfaction and a feeling that reorganization was necessary.

During 1937 and 1937 the hospital's trustees and medical staff wrested with the problems caused by overcrowding and need for up-to-date accommodations for the technological advances in surgery and rehabilitation.

Finally, a consultant summoned for advice examined the hospital's corporate structure as well as its physical plant, pronouncing both unsound. Tamblyn and Brown, of New York City, hired to advise on a possible capital funds drive, wisely placed the problem where it belonged, back in the hands of the community, with the recommendation that a committee of nine citizens study the organizational structure of the hospital. It would be interesting to know who recommended the chairmanship of James Langley. The rest of the committee was equally politic consisting of trustees Mary Wood, Mrs. Harry Lake and Mrs. Albert Ordway, citizens Grace Hanus, I. Reed Gourley, and Rufus Weston, and, from the medical staff, Drs. Gerard Gaudrault and Clarence Butterfield.

Their report, dated January 1938, called for a corporate reorganization and a new set of by-laws.[5] It explained that the hospital had, since 1930, been operating under the assumption that merely by saying so it had become a general hospital. While it is true that a vote of trustees had been taken in 1935 to change the by-laws and the name, nothing legal had actually taken place. Technically the institution remained a hospital for women and children, a potential source of embarrassment to trustees. The legality of monetary bequests to such an entity was in question.

The report's recommendations, incorporating those made by Tamblyn and Brown, were consolidated into four general policies: that New Hampshire Memorial Hospital (is practically and) should continue to be a general hospital. Steps should be taken to make this a legal fact and that the board of trustees be reorganized to fully recognize the existing and future general hospital policy and the delimitation of the area which the hospital actually serves. The efficiency of the physical plant should be improved by provision of additional facilities which will best serve the general hospital policy of the institution. Finally, plans should be prepared for improvements of the plant and that cost of the improvements be determined before concentrated efforts are made to finance them through a limited solicitation of friends of the hospital.

The committee justified each recommendation stating emphatically that their paramount concern was the order in which they were approached. It is doubtful that the trustees expected such an overwhelming condemnation of their organizational structure, for that is what the report in its now faded green binder was. Fortunately it also presented a careful plan of reorganization approved by legal counsel, and, what was ultimately more important, it recommended the recruitment of more men, community leaders, as trustees.

By the time all of these areas had been addressed, James Langley was at the helm of a more businesslike organization which began to streamline its operation. Stocks paying no dividends were sold. Langley urged the city to pay individual hospital bills for city cases rather than grant an annual appropriation. Committee responsibilities, redefined, accomplished more work outside monthly board meetings, shortening those sessions appreciably.

One note of humanity softened the brisk tone of the new board. Dr. Ellen Wallace, now president emeritus of the board and retired from active practice, was invited to make the hospital her home for the rest of her life as a gesture of appreciation for her many years of devotion to the institution. She accepted in a gracefully worded note to the trustees and occupied the Jane Hapgood room for five years, attending board meetings and retaining her interest in the hospital's work. She died there in 1945 at the age of 92.

Both hospitals were functioning efficiently by the beginning of the forties, each with a hard working board that did not hesitate to cooperate with the other for the welfare of the community, but there were occasional lapses, one occurring in 1935 that serves as an illustration:

Margaret Pillsbury's trustees became convinced that their hospital should have a closed staff, not closed to the application of additional physicians, but closed in the sense that physician members of its staff would not be allowed to serve on the staffs of other hospitals. Their belief in this idea was derived from their understanding of new organizational standards then being promulgated by the American College of Surgeons.

Naturally, they informed Memorial's board of trustees of their impending decision, causing near panic on South Spring Street. Physicians must determine which hospital they would serve and most concluded that Pillsbury, the larger of the two, having a more diverse patient population and better facilities, would be the better choice. Memorial was faced with the prospect of losing virtually its entire staff.

When Pillsbury's trustees tabled the motion to pass this amendment to its by-laws pending a survey of hospital needs in Concord, Memorial's trustees asked to meet with a like group from the other hospital. In the meantime common sense prevailed. Mrs. James Remick, president of Memorial's board, organizer of its Hospital Associates and president of the New Hampshire Federation of Women's Clubs, went to the source of the problem. For a clarification of the intent of the American College, she telephoned its president in Boston.

One can almost sense the amusement in his reply that this closed staff was recommended only for big city hospitals of 200 beds or more to improve service to patients. Why, hospitals in a small community such as Concord would want to work together, sharing their roles in patient care. Evidently this explanation satisfied both parties; the closed staff was not mentioned again. One year later the vote, which apparently had been taken, became a source of embarassment to Pillsbury's trustees. Memorial Hospital's annual report revealed that many of Concord's physicians had not felt free to serve on Memorial's staff and at the same time be on the active staff of the Pillsbury Hospital. Even though Memorial's trustees had received assurances that the vote would not be enforced, it resulted in bad feelings on the part of Memorial's board because they had been carrying out their work with only five physicians. The publicity given the issue probably did more good than harm, for it assured Pillsbury's doctors that the vote was not binding.[6]

7

Graduates Before 1940
and the War Years

hen the phase-out of the Concord Hospital School of Nursing was announced in the fall of 1986 and planning for this volume began, alumni of the three schools were notified through their newsletter of the closing. The school and the author received a number of letters from older graduates who volunteered memorabilia and memories of their school days.

It would have been exciting to hear from a member of that first class of the Margaret Pillsbury School or from the young women who served in World War I in France. At the time of the hospital's fiftieth anniversary in 1934, it was noted that graduates were eligible to practice in any state in the union or any foreign country without further examination owing to the school's recent approval by the New York State Board of Regents. It was the first school in New Hampshire to be so approved and graduates were, indeed, found throughout the continent. Lilian Streeter noted in her chronicle of the school's history that a graduate (whom she did not name) had just taken charge of a department of the University of Southern California, while another (Wilhelmina R. Ley, 1908), a member of the Episcopal Order of St. Ann, was accomplishing much good in settlement work in the slums of Boston. She described the hospital mission in Alaska maintained by the Protestant Episcopal Missions of America where for several years a member of the class of 1924, Addie Gavel, ministered to the Indians. Arriving at Fort Yukon with one other nurse during an influenza epidemic, it was three months before they were joined by a physician. Gavel traveled by dog sled

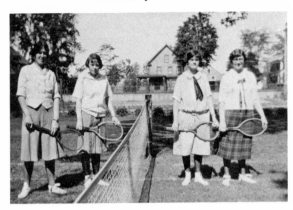

A grass court on the grounds of Memorial Hospital furnished off-duty exercise for these doubles players in 1927. Basketball was another sport popular with student nurses at that time.

covering thousands of miles, practicing both medicine and nursing.[1]

Fortunately, although the experiences of these earliest graduates are lost to us, several alumnae of the twenties and thirties have taken the time to set down their memories for us. Here is the account of Ruth Inman (Tozier) of her years of training and beyond, in her own words.

The class of 1929 came to the Margaret Pillsbury General Hospital in Sept. 1926. We were housed in one of two houses at the corner of South Main and Maitland Streets. The other house was for the help.

As probationers our uniforms were medium blue with well starched white aprons and collars. After three months we were given the bibs, cuffs and caps, starched like the aprons. Our caps were made of handkerchief linen. Seniors were given narrow black velvet bands for their caps. Later we had navy blue wool capes lined with red wool and the letters MPGH on the stand-up collars.

Our hours were 7 A.M. to 7 P.M. with two hours off to study, classes etc., each day, one half day a week off A.M. or P.M. The probationers went on duty every A.M. with the older students and learned while helping until their class time.

Our instructress was a wonderful person, teacher, and counselor, Miss McNeven. She was a Canadian nurse, had served overseas in World War I. She stayed with us about a year when the new superintendent came. That is another story.

The new nurses' home was built in 1927 and 1928. The annex was added with twelve private rooms on each floor, medical and surgical on the first floor and obstetrical on the second with the nursery.

The attic of the old building was made into a large operating room. (It had been on the first floor, Pillsbury St. side, by the ambulance door), two delivery rooms, work room where dressings were made, autoclave room. A new elevator was installed from the basement at the front entrance. A covered corridor was built from the annex to serve the basement, first and second floors to the elevator. The second floor of the corridor was a ramp which meant the obstetrical patients had to be pushed on a stretcher up a grade to the elevator and then to the delivery room, no small job if the patient was in labor.

The laundry was in the basement near the heating system. A laundry building was built beside Maitland Street with the heating system below it and a tall smokestack beside it. A tunnel was dug from the laundry to the basement of the old building with a cement cover on it. This was nice when we could go under cover from the basement of the home. The classrooms were on the ground floor of the nurses' home beneath the nurses' rooms. Such a change from the old house. The nurses' rooms were all single. We moved in in 1928.

We had our children's training at Boston Dispensary on Beech Street. It was my bad luck to catch diphtheria while working in the clinic. I was taken via ambulance to the Boston City Hospital contagion ward. I was the only one there.

There was a separate contagious ward near the Margaret Pillsbury we called the pest house.

Our psychiatry training consisted of lectures at the State Hospital, now the New Hampshire Hospital, by Dr. Dolloff, the superintendent. He would bring in patients as examples of his topic. Also, we saw some patients in tubs with canvas covers and warm running water. This was a treatment.

We had gym exercises at the Kimball School once a week in the evening. We walked there which was exercise enough. Our transportation up-town was by trolley car. They went by the front of the hospital to the car barns in the Boston & Maine railroad repair shops across the street. Buses eventually took their place.

We were not allowed to call the nurses or doctors by any name but their last name with Miss or Dr. before it. That later became [the use of] just the last name.

The most exciting event that happened was when Charles Lindbergh was paraded down Main Street in an auto. He came down So. Main Street to Pillsbury Street where he stopped and handed a bouquet of red, white and blue flowers to someone. We knew he would be coming so all who could, nurses and patients were out to greet him. I had a red rose from the center [of the bouquet].

There were no graduation exercises until the late 1930s. We were handed our diploma or had to ask for it. Mine was handed to me by a supervisor when I asked for it. The superintendent was in Boston.

In 1938 when the valley was flooded so high and electricity was out everywhere, the National Guard brought in two units (generators) to supply enough electricity for the operating and delivery rooms in the old building and the annex with lights and the elevators. That lasted for several weeks.[2]

Mrs. Tozier remembered, in an afterthought, that Dr. Fred Eveleth taught students to take x-ray pictures of minor cases and that some became quite proficient. Ruth Allen (1912) became his assistant, keeping his records. Instructresses who influenced her, in addition to Miss McNeven, were Superintendent Mary Whittaker, Mrs. VanPelt, and Agnes Joyce. Two members of the class preceding her gave her a great deal of assistance. They were Caroline Oldham (Stickney) and Wilda Torrance (Little).

Genevieve Mullen (McDonald) wrote to tell us about her years at Margaret Pillsbury. The circumstances surrounding her graduation are intriguing for she graduated two weeks later than she expected to owing to confusion with a classmate who resembled her. Mullen was charged with a two week illness suffered by her classmate, receiving her pin from a nursing supervisor in December 1932. She was involved in virtually all forms of nursing during her long career: floor and private duty, x-ray nurse, physician's office nurse and finally, work with the New Hampshire Division of Public Health as nurse-coordinator of preschool vision and hearing. In her Florida retirement years she has served as a volunteer school nurse for a private school.

Genevieve Mullen's stream-of-consciousness memories of her training:

Starch — cuffs and little round collar cutting into neck — black shoes and stockings — hairnets — always hungry. Six weeks spent in isolation ward (pest house) on Pillsbury Street, boiling dishes, glasses, utensils. Laundry soaked in Lysol and then the hand wringing so ole Mike could deposit in laundry. My parents upset as they could not comprehend this as nursing. Their baby girl after five boys subject to this treatment. "Come home" in all the mail. I ignored their pleas to come home. I had to prove to my five brothers I would make it as they had bets together and vowed I would run home when things got difficult. They forgot my Irish background, no matter how rough, always do the best you can.[3]

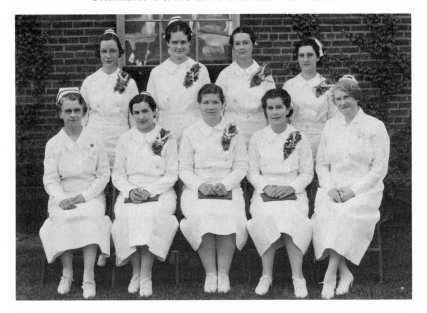

*Memorial Hospital's class of 1936 poses on graduation day
with its instructor and Superintendent Cleland.*

Emma Werner (Winslow) who also lives in Concord, appears in the snap-
shot of an apron-clad group of ten probationers entering Memorial's training school in 1927, to emerge three years later diminished by three. She has
presented her red-lined navy wool cape to the growing collection of nursing memorabilia awaiting cataloging for display.

If one picture is worth a thousand words, then the scrapbook sent by Ph.D
nursing education consultant Vurlyne Ellsworth (Boan) celebrating the years
1936 to 1939 at Margaret Pillsbury's school must be worth volumes, for it
portrays in glorious black and white three years of moments snatched from
classes, floor duty and affiliations to record the lighter moments of a nurse's
education. Vurlyne, who lives in Arizona now, first appears with classmates
in the uniform of the probationer, two months later introducing each with
a newly coined nickname. "Poil," "Butch," and "Slug" are capped in early 1937,
go on to summer vacations and are seen next in operating room regalia. During the summer of 1938 they attend the annual party given by chief surgeon
James Jameson at his vacation home. Fall 1938 finds the young women in
New York City for an affiliation in medicine and pediatrics at Bellevue

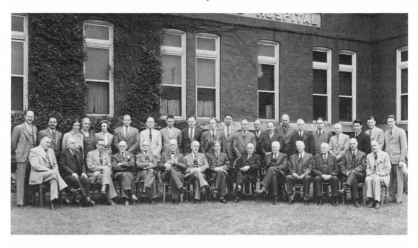

Some members of the medical staff were new in 1939 when they gathered for this portrait out-side Margaret Pillsbury Hospital. John Branson is sixth from left in the back row, J. Dunbar Shields third from right. Clinton Mullins is at extreme left in the back row. The early days are represented by surgeon emeritus Chancey Adams (holding cat in front row) and dentist William Young, second from left in front row.

Hospital. The pictures here show rows of white iron cribs and small solemn faces. They find time to snap each other at the traditional sites, Rockefeller Center, Fifth Avenue's Pulaski Day parade, posed beside the lions at the New York Public Library.

Back to New Hampshire and another picnic with the surgical staff. There is a Christmas card photo of the doctors in front of the entrance to the hospital signed by them and by the nursing and administrative staff. The album ends with wedding pictures and, considering the times, a couple of uniformed poses. Eight probationers entered school at 2:00 P.M. on September 8, 1936. Three left during the next two years. Five graduated at various times during 1939, having made up clinical hours lost to illness.

Such are the memories of the years between the wars, memories of long days, strict obedience to superiors, horseplay during leisure hours, scenes from the innocent era that ended abruptly on December 7, 1941.

The war years in Concord were like those across the country. There were shortages of food and clothing, of tires and durable goods, but primarily of manpower. Pillsbury was stretched beyond its limit to care for patients while upholding standards of cleanliness and concern for patients' wellbeing. The children's ward, needing more nurses than adult wards, was closed in 1944. Operating rooms could be used only during the week.

Trustees enlisted the aid of chapter members to handle some of the housekeeping tasks for which employees were unavailable. Mrs. Gardner Emmons, president of the auxiliary in 1944, was requested to organize a group of women to assist in washing dishes, dusting, dry mopping, and setting up trays.

Still active in the community in her eighth decade, Abbie Emmons remembers those days well. "I mopped the floors of the men's ward," she recalls. She found ten or twelve women who were able to help, including her sister-in-law Margaret Emmons, an active trustee who was assigned to the operating room after a little training. Margaret told Abbie that one day she was handed an amputated leg for disposal, no doubt an unforgettable experience for the uninitiated.[4]

In retrospect, this group of women epitomized the wartime attitude prevalent throughout the nation. Though they were accustomed to household help themselves and making do at home without aid, such social leaders as Rose White Winship, Mary Louise DeLahunta, and Abbie and Margaret Emmons pitched in with a will to help the hospital their families and friends had founded.

Margaret Pillsbury's medical staff was reduced by sixteen physicians in 1942. Of those on the staff then who served in the armed forces during World War II, we are fortunate to have a number who live in retirement in the Concord area: Warren Butterfield, Philip Forsberg, J. Dunbar Shields, and Ellsworth Tracy. Those who are no longer with us include physicians Donald Barton, John Branson, Eugene Chamberlain, Carl Dahlgren, Raymond Galloway, MacLean Gill, Thomas Halligan, Joseph McCarthy, J. Kenneth McLeod, Alfred Mihachik, and dentists William Young, Jr. and Harlan Besse.

For the first time a businessman, Fred A. Sharp, was at the administrative helm at Margaret Pillsbury. In fact, Sharp was the first man to run the institution and the first to bear the title administrator. He had been comptroller of the New York Hospital for some years and executive director of the White Plains Hospital for the preceding three years. It was noted in 1942's annual report that Sharp had come to the hospital in time (January 1941) to oversee the operation under normal circumstances before the upheaval caused by the war. He followed Mary Whittaker, R.N. whose seventeen year superintendency had been the longest to date and who, by all accounts, was beloved by students, staff, and patients. Sharp's business experience proved invaluable in guiding the hospital through the difficult war years when economies of all kinds were practiced, some ordered by the government, some self-inflicted. Everyone over the age of fifty remembers shortages of food items, most prominently sugar and butter. How many remember the government directive prohibiting the slicing of bread by bakeries? Jane and Michael Stern's book *Square Meals* recalls this silly regulation for us along with the meatless, fatless, sometimes flavorless recipes housewives fed hungry war workers and children exhausted from rolling tin foil into balls and hoeing the victory gardens.[5] Multiply individual economies by a score and one might approximate the enormity of the task accomplished by hospital trustees and staff as they attempted to carry out the old directive "Eat it up, wear it out, make it do or do without." One of the "do withouts" was the costly annual report for 1941, omitted for the first time in the hospital's history.

It was impossible to do without nurses. Those under forty who could be spared joined the armed forces. Young women were not entering the nursing schools in sufficient numbers to meet the greatly expanded needs of hospitals. Competition from the women's auxiliaries of the armed services and from well-paid industrial jobs attracted many away from the strenuous training required of student nurses. A plan to educate more student nurses was badly needed.

Such a plan evolved from legislation introduced by Congresswoman Frances Payne Bolton, a Republican from Ohio. Building on earlier legislation she had sponsored that made federal money available for scholarships, additional teachers, and expanded clinical facilities, the new bill aimed at increasing enrollment in schools of nursing, accelerating the training period to include full-time service in civilian, military, public health, veterans' and Indian hospitals during the last six months.

Inaugurated in March 1943, the United States Cadet Corps would train over 169,000 students during its six-year existence. Margaret Pillsbury's school of nursing was accepted as a unit of the Cadet Corps on November 1, 1943; New Hampshire Memorial joined during 1944.[6]

There are few mysteries surrounding the Cadet Corps since we are in possession of a complete set of records of a scope that only the United States government could require. The amount of red tape wrapped firmly around the smallest move on the part of a member unit is remarkable, the work required of school administrators unending, but we learn much about the schools, their students, and curricula during the forties from these documents. The corps was run by the Division of Nurse Education of the U.S. Public Health Service. Its chief was Lucille Petry, on the nurse education staff for two years and recently appointed dean of Cornell University's New York Hospital School of Nursing. Responsible to the Surgeon General, Petry was assisted by an advisory committee on the training of nurses. She and

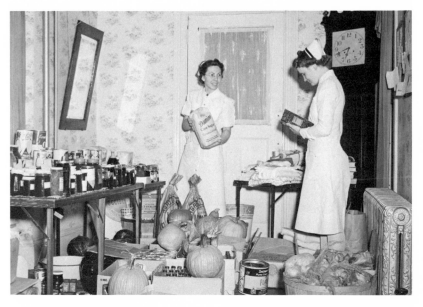

A contribution is recorded following a bounteous harvest on Donation Day. For many years, Margaret Pillsbury's annual report acknowledged every donation.

her staff succeeded in exceeding the enrollment quotas they established of 65,000 during the first 12 months, 60,000 the following year.

Under the Bolton Act training was accelerated from thirty-six months to thirty. In order to get around the state board stipulations that training should last thirty-six months, a compromise arrived at a three-level progression. During the first nine months in school while a student studied the basic sciences and nursing fundamentals, she was designated a pre-cadet. Junior cadets were students during the next fifteen to twenty-one months of clinical training. The senior cadet had actually completed her training, but state boards demanded the extra six months and this was the period during which the student undertook a practice assignment in her home hospital or in another civilian, military, veterans', or government institution.

Most schools had the participation of 80 to 100 percent of their students, the advertising was glamorous promising "a lifetime education free." Not the least of the enticements, in addition to a $15 to $30 monthly stipend as they progressed, were the handsome uniforms designed for the Corps by Mollie Parnis with a jaunty beret by Sally Victor. Though the school's student uniform was worn in the hospital, the Cadet uniform with its matching reefer

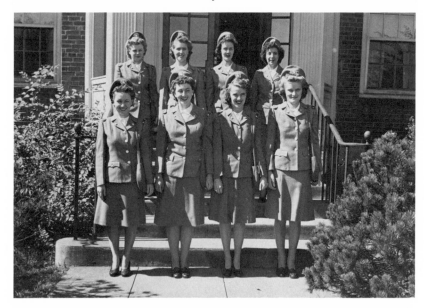

Students show off their Cadet uniforms on the steps of the nurses' residence at Margaret Pillsbury Hospital. Margaret Mitchell (Wallace), class of 1945 who later became an instructor in the Concord Hospital School is second from right in the first row.

coat or raincoat was de rigeur on the street. There was a smart grey and white striped summer version as well and the photographs of Pillsbury and Memorial students so attired shine with the pride they must have felt.

Back in the office of the director all was not so rosy. Folder after folder of correspondence and monthly reports, as well as requisition forms for textbooks and uniforms testify to the complexity of administering such a program. Schools were visited by the Division of Nurse Education to evaluate the quality of their educational and clinical offerings as well as the efficiency of the administration of the program. A letter to Anne Shepard, director of Memorial Hospital's school in 1944, makes specific recommendations to improve the organizational aspects as well as its educational facilities. A clear picture of New England thrift emerges from this suggestion to the director:

Your own responsibilities are too important and time consuming for you to carry them without at least a secretary if not an assistant, especially since you teach three subjects, take care of the students' health and do a great deal of clerical work in addition to carrying your other duties as Director of the school.

From this series of recommendations came the nucleus of the school we know today. A faculty organization was outlined to study problems of curriculum, student welfare, and continuing education for faculty. Postgraduate education was recommended for faculty and the director. It was suggested that the students' library be removed from a classroom and given a room of its own in the nurses' residence. Most prominent among recommendations was the request to reduce the student workload to forty-eight hours per week including class time and to eliminate night duty during the precadet period, a task that apparently was underway at the time of the visit.

The senior cadet assignment proved particularly difficult to handle during the years of the Corps. While there were many assignments students wanted to take, often an ancillary problem such as lack of housing at the host site or a vacation due the student intervened. Sometimes the sheer necessity of retaining the student at her home hospital prevented her from accepting an assignment half a continent away. The correspondence concerning these assignments indicates that not many students were able to work in exotic, far-off places, a circumstance that prevailed nationally. Statistics reveal that 73 percent of the senior cadets remained in their home hospitals for the duration of their service in the Corps. Actually, marriage and the desire to follow a serviceman husband prevented many students from even finishing their training.

Because both Concord schools were struggling to achieve the levels of educational quality demanded of Cadet Corps participation, they began to cooperate with each other to some degree. They were located, handily, a few blocks from each other. Hazel Harris, a longtime housemother, was living in the neighborhood then, a cook for the Margaret Pillsbury Hospital. She remembers seeing the students walking between the two schools for lectures, the first area of cooperation. The lectures given by physicians were consolidated to avoid wasting the valuable time of wartime's overworked practitioners. Margaret Pillsbury lost its science instructor to a large university, and in order to obtain a well-qualified instructor, appealed to Colby Junior College (now Colby-Sawyer College). In 1941 Memorial Hospital had been granted use of the Concord High School laboratory and its instructor, a Mr. Dodge, to teach chemistry to student nurses. During these years students shared their classrooms at both schools with the large groups of Red Cross nurses aides who were being trained throughout the country to augment nursing staffs.

Both hospitals weathered the war years efficiently, aided immeasurably by the advent of health insurance. Blue Cross had come on the scene in the late thirties in time to keep hospitals in action during the depression. Its increasing popularity did much to fill beds during the war years.

The old saying about the ill wind that blows some good can surely be applied to the effects of the war on nursing education and, as we now know, on the evolution of health care, particularly surgical advancements and the development of life-saving drug therapies. Physicians and nurses who returned from war service in the mid-forties had grown in skill and experience, qualities that contributed in great measure to hospital care's technological growth, war's legacy to an expanding postwar population.

8

Anatomy of a Merger

ames McLellan Langley was born in Hyde Park, Massachusetts, in 1894, a Dartmouth graduate and a captain in the infantry during World War I. He came to Concord in 1923 after a five year stint as a reporter on the *Manchester Union-Leader* to take charge of the newly consolidated *Concord Daily Monitor* and the daily *New Hampshire Patriot*. Said to be painfully shy in the early days, he may have immersed himself in community activities to lose that shyness. If so, he was more than successful shedding not only his reticence but his first wife as he worked his way through nearly a score of boards, commissions and committees, many of them aimed at the modernization of health care delivery in New Hampshire.[1]

Even during the period of the merger Langley was looking at health care with what today's jargon would term the "global view." Prepaid hospital, medical, and surgical bills became a reality in New Hampshire when he founded and headed a Blue Cross chapter and served as a director of Blue Shield. He headed the commission sponsoring legislation to license hospitals and other health facilities and was instrumental in securing enabling legislation to take advantage of Hill-Burton funds for hospital construction in New Hampshire.

The story of the merger begins shortly after Langley's reorganization of Memorial Hospital's corporate structure during which it had become apparent to him that Concord would be better served by one institution. His first salvo was a letter to Pillsbury's board in February 1939 proposing a sur-

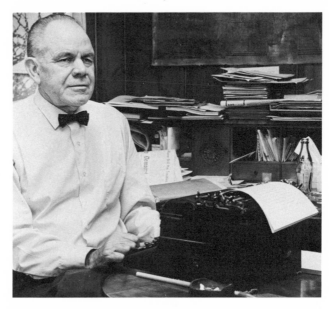

James McLellan Langley, editor and publisher of the Concord Monitor
*and architect of the merger which created Concord Hospital. This photo
was taken at his desk not long before his death in 1968.*

vey of both hospitals to "ascertain the advisability of combining the institutions for the best interests of the citizens of Concord." The survey was approved by Pillsbury's trustees, and a Dr. Pollock, whose credentials are un-
fortunately lost to posterity, agreed to carry out the work. The results appear
to have favored consolidation but the report was not made part of either
hospital's records. The public-spirited doctor would accept only $10 of the
$100 offered him by the two groups.

Inexplicably, the move for consolidation was abandoned in June 1941 and
national events which followed made further work on this project difficult.
Throughout the upheaval created by the war the citizens who managed the
city's hospitals were able to continue their activities without interruption.
Fortunately most were beyond the age of active military service, and many
were women who combined duties as Red Cross Gray Ladies with their
trusteeships and advisory committees. Many were learning for the first time
of the joys of maintaining large houses without the maids and cooks who
had gone off to war along with the family chauffeurs.

Initially, formal consolidation efforts were put off while the two boards struggled with problems created by the war. These people were adept at stretching dollars with skills honed during the Depression, but employees were harder to stretch and it gradually dawned on them that activities common to both institutions could be combined for a saving of man hours, an idea that advanced the cause of merger immeasurably. If lectures could be given to both groups of students at once then laundry might be done for both hospitals at one location and perhaps only one maternity department was needed.

A second legacy of the Depression was the postponement of necessary maintenance and modernization at both locations so that balanced budgets could be presented to trustees. Plans to catch up were thwarted by the war leaving both hospitals with antiquated facilities.

Fred Sharp recommended $10,000 worth of purchases and improvements in his report to the Pillsbury board in April, 1941 with priorities identified as "rush," "as soon as possible," "June or July," and "near future." The next year $155,000 of construction work was undertaken to correct deficiencies in the building which was now over fifty years old. Memorial's problems were similar. They had shored up the old wooden structure on South Street, having endured overcrowding in the newer South Spring Street structure while the work was in progress. Both boards anticipated bad times ahead.

Although there are no indications in the official records of either hospital between June 1941 and December 1944 that a merger was contemplated, probably a great deal of planning was occurring behind the scenes. In January 1944 Pillsbury's Board President Benjamin Couch explained a proposal for a new hospital to be called Concord Hospital which would be built from funds obtained from the sale of the two existing hospitals and from federal funds thought to be obtainable after the war. He asked for volunteers among the trustees who would be willing to serve as incorporators of the new institution. Couch joined women trustees Hollis, Swenson, Dolloff, and Messrs. McSwiney, Banks, Jenkins, Everett, and Tilton. These people and others met at the Concord Chamber of Commerce office on October 17, 1944, to sign the articles of agreement. Benjamin W. Couch presided; Laurence Duncan was elected temporary clerk.

Thirty-five men and women (for the record, eleven women, twenty-four men) were unanimously elected members of the corporation and the same group was nominated and unanimously elected trustees. James Langley became president and Laurence Duncan secretary.[2]

On October 31 the executive committee of the new corporation met, probably wondering where to begin, but Langley was ready with a pamphlet

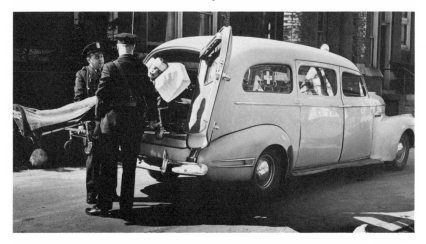

Past and present are sharply contrasted in these two photos. Above, police transfer a patient from the department's ambulance to the Pillsbury Hospital in the late forties.

called "Making Better Health Available to All" prepared for small hospitals facing consolidation. It recommended that problems be solved in the following order: Select a site for the new hospital, prepare building plans, then obtain funds for the project. Using city maps they quickly identified a tract of land on Pleasant Street which was in part owned by the Shawmut Realty Trust. They recorded, at that first meeting, pledges to the building fund from I. Reed Gourley, Dr. Pierre Boucher, and the Monitor Patriot Company.

A month later, the full board voted to purchase or acquire options on lands owned by Shawmut, the Christian Science Pleasant View Home, Sadie Dunstane, Margaret Ford, and George W. Hill, north of Pleasant Street and west of Grandview Avenue. Langley would have been familiar with the tract since he lived nearly adjacent to it at 278 Pleasant Street. He described the fifty-acre site to the group in December explaining that it would cost about $20,000. Ironically, in view of the intended purpose for the land, it was also a historic site where a granite monument had been erected in 1837 in memory of Samuel Bradley, Jonathan Bradley, Obadiah Peters, John Bean, and John Lufkin who were massacred by the Indians on August 11, 1746, near the spot. Options for nearly all parcels had been obtained and with a new pledge of $10,000 from Rumford Printing Company added to the Monitor's gift, the land could be purchased.

By February 1945 the firm of Coolidge, Shepley, Bulfinch and Abbott, of Boston, had been selected to draw up preliminary plans. In April the board

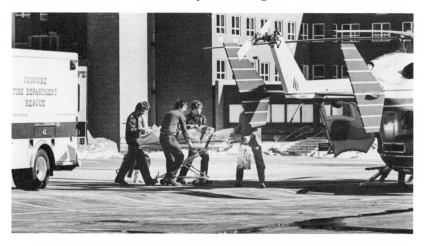

Transfer of a critically ill patient by the fire department's emergency medical technicians, with portable life-saving equipment in place, to a waiting helicopter for a flight to Boston.

voted to allow Margaret Ford to occupy her cottage house on the property until they were ready to sell or move it.

In October a legal opinion advised that a merger of the two existing hospitals would be required before a fund drive could be initiated on behalf of the new institution. The court must be petitioned for permission to transfer assets of the two hospitals to Concord Hospital. The executive committee was authorized to employ a director to oversee the operation of the two hospitals. Fred Sharp had submitted his resignation when he saw that merger was imminent.

The request for petition to the Superior Court of Merrimack County appeared in the *Monitor's* legal notices in March 1946 and the decree was issued by Judge John H. Leahy on May 7, 1946, directing Margaret Pillsbury and Memorial Hospitals to transfer all property to Concord Hospital which was authorized to hold and administer such property. The article that announced the decree also stated that N. Conant Faxon had been employed to direct the new hospital beginning on June 17. Faxon was then assistant superintendent of the Cambridge Hospital, a 272-bed institution with a more than 200-student school of nursing. His wife was a graduate nurse. If these credentials were not recommendation enough, the article revealed that the new director was a Harvard graduate and the son of Dr. N.W. Faxon, director of Massachusetts General Hospital.

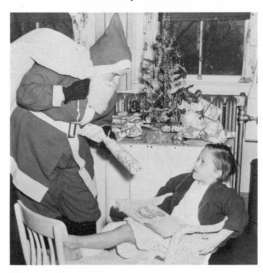

*Santa delivers a package to a young convalescent in
Pillsbury Hospital's Bancroft-Sullivan ward in 1948.*

With the help of an advance from the hospital, Faxon and his family settled in at 5 Grandview Avenue, a desirable vantage point from which to oversee what trustees assumed was the imminent construction of a new hospital.[3] His first duties, though, were to consolidate the two nursing schools,
hiring replacements for the nurses who had been in charge both in the hospitals and as instructors in the schools. Accounting systems were standardized
in both institutions and a common rate schedule was created to assure that
each hospital was charging the same price for similar accommodations. The
medical staff appointed committees to represent each unit. Their first task
became the correction of deficiencies named in the most recent American
College of Surgeons survey.

   Those who were appointed to the first nursing school committee were
Helen Pelren, Natt Burbank, Florence Clark, Grace Stevens, Mae Kenney,
and Dr. Thomas Dudley. The first class to enter the new school numbered
thirteen when they began training in September 1946, possibly an unlucky
number for them as only four remained to graduate in September 1949. It
is unclear about the classes that entered both schools before the merger, but
graduated after it. Apparently they were considered graduates of the pre-
existing schools. Graduates are listed for all three schools for 1947. By 1948
Concord Hospital School of Nursing was the diploma-granting authority.

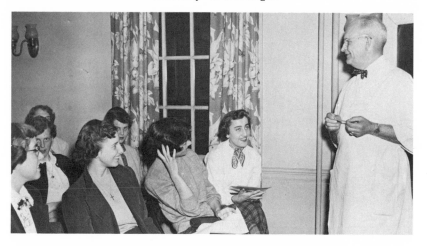

Dr. James Park, the hospital's pathologist, has clearly charmed these St. John's High School students as he describes "Careers in a Hospital," a recruiting effort in 1952.

At the conclusion of the war the merger of hospitals and schools was nearly accomplished, but if Conant Faxon thought he could concentrate on plans for the new building he was greatly mistaken, for the view from Grandview Avenue would remain undarkened by Langley's vision during Faxon's tenure at Concord Hospital.

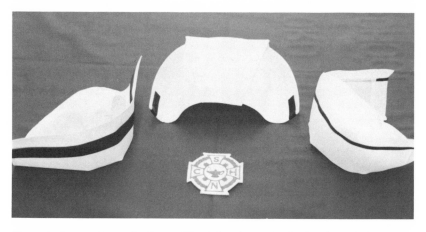

The cap in the center is worn by Concord Hospital graduates who developed a symbolic meaning for each of its six buttons. At left is Memorial Hospital's cap, at right the one worn by Pillsbury Hospital graduates. Male graduates wear the emblem of the School on the left shoulder of the uniform tunic.

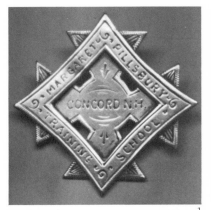

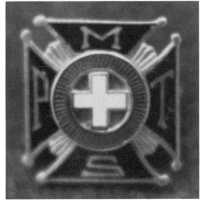

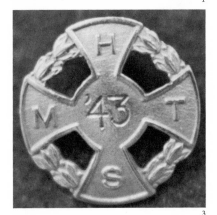

The first Pillsbury pin (1) was of sterling silver, made and donated by the W.B. Durgin Company, and the second (2) was designed sometime after 1920 and worn until the merger. The Memorial pin (3) had the student's year of graduation engraved at its center. The oval pin (4) was the first designed for the new Concord Hospital School and was replaced shortly thereafter by the one in use today (5).

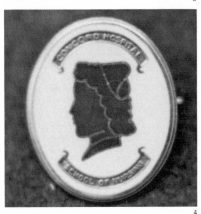

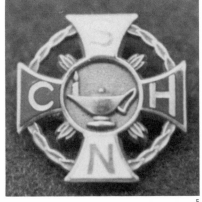

9

Frustrations and Accomplishments

im Langley's helpful little pamphlet listed the third step in the consolidation process as "obtain funds." The trustees had seen this process as essentially a simple one. They would mount a community-wide campaign to raise the funds needed over and above those gained from the sale of the two hospital properties and the funds to be appropriated by a government eager to contribute to the improvement of health care facilities made inadequate by a burgeoning post-war population. That they were wrong in this estimation of the task was not early evident. Langley explained to the public in a *Monitor* editorial on May 8, 1946, that it would be impossible to build and occupy a new hospital before 1948 and that Margaret Pillsbury and Memorial Hospitals would be operated under the new director much as they were functioning then. He estimated that preliminary plans could be completed by January 1, 1947, but working drawings could consume a year in preparation, the building process another year.

Not taken into consideration by anyone was the enormity of the task of maintaining the antiquated Pillsbury and Memorial properties, of securing and paying staff, of educating and housing students, of planning, running, and paying for a fund drive and architects' fees, all the while dealing with the effects of World War II and ultimately the Korean conflict. Patient stays in hospitals were reduced by half between 1941 and 1951. Penicillin, introduced to Concord for hospital use in 1944 and streptomycin a year or so later, bore a great share of the responsibility for this as did the new techniques and instrumentation of surgery. Prepaid medical insurance was be-

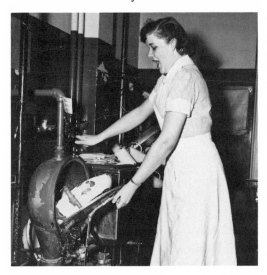

*Exploring the mysteries of the bedpan flusher, the fresh-
man student gets an unexpected shower in this scene from
the last days of the old Pillsbury Hospital.*

ginning to change the way people used hospitals, making greater demands
on them. The trustees had no ability to predict these changes which created a hindrance to their multi-million dollar building program.

We are ahead of our story, for these problems did not become evident
until after the fund drive. On May 25, 1946, city planner Gustave Lehtinen
was shown in the *Monitor* with artist Arch McDonnell admiring the newly
created model of the proposed building built from preliminary plans which
included a four-story nursing school and nurses residence. A community
relations committee of the trustees headed by Gardner Tilton was conducting a survey of local residents to determine the level of satisfaction with
health care in Concord. They were rewarded with a 96 percent response indicating that both hospitals were overcrowded and inadequate. Eighty-eight
percent of those responding said that, were they able, they would leave money to a hospital in Concord.

Heartened by this overwhelming confidence in their project the trustees
released the architectural drawings from which the model had been created. The structure had a central seven-story core from which radiated four
wings. No luxury was omitted including air-conditioning for surgical and
obstetrical suites. Four dining rooms had been designed for staff and em-

ployees of the new building, to have a 40 percent greater capacity (221 beds, 36 bassinets) than the two existing units. It was expected to cost $1,700,000.

The plan was for the fund drive to raise a million dollars, the rest to come from federal, state, and municipal sources. A citizens' committee of 250 dined at the Eagle Hotel on September 17 to hear the project described by James Langley. Gardner Tilton, Mayor Charles Davie, and Dr. Carleton Metcalf, then secretary of the New Hampshire Medical Society, were additional speakers.

The public campaign was to begin on January 27, 1947, but the *Monitor* immediately began to herald large initial gifts in order to whet the appetites of its readers for the memorial possibilities of such largess. One could ensure a favorable public image with a generous donation to such a universally approved cause. Trustees themselves and their families pledged over $150,000, many designating specific units to be established by their gifts. Thirty-eight members of the medical staff contributed $124,500.

Frank Sulloway, treasurer of the hospital corporation was in charge of these memorial gifts aided by Harry G. Emmons. They used a brochure entitled "The New Concord Hospital," illustrated with detailed floor plans and a schedule of opportunities for "creative memorials."[1] A twenty-four-month installment plan was offered for the payment of pledges which described the cost of the building's entire ground floor as six equal payments of $22,150. Three types of semi-private rooms could be had for $3,600, $4,200 and $4,800, or using the six-payment plan, $600, $700 and $800. Student rooms in the adjacent nursing school building were $2,100 each, the biochemistry laboratory could be dedicated for $8,400. More than forty of Concord's leading citizens, most of them lawyers and physicians, served on the committee soliciting these major gifts.

Meanwhile, in an effort to secure every possible source of funds, the trustees asked the Superior Court of Merrimack County to petition the State Director of Trust Funds Ernest D'Amours on behalf of the hospital to change payment to a beneficiary of the will of E. Smith Tenney, late owner of the Tenney Coal Company. He had willed his housekeeper $100 a month for life, and after one other bequest the remainder of the estate, nearly $400,000 would come to the hospital. In order to speed the process D'Amours asked for the authority to purchase an annuity to take care of the housekeeper's legacy. His petition called the hospital "a pressing public need."

The Langley family's own gift, $24,000 from James M. and Marcia Langley and Esther Newell, would build and equip the first floor kitchen. The dedicatees were Frank E. and Mary B. Langley, parents of the donors. In accepting the gift Frank Sulloway commented on the appropriate recognition of the keen interest of the elder Langleys in "community health as influenced by adequate hospitals." Frank E. Langley had been a founder of the Barre City Hospital in Vermont and was its president at his death in 1938.[2]

The Margaret Pillsbury Chapter chose a private room for their $5,100 contribution honoring Gladys Dolloff their founder and first president. The organization numbered 250 women in 1946 before merging with Memorial Hospital's auxiliary to become the Concord Hospital Associates.

The next group to begin work concentrated its approaches to some four hundred citizens whose gifts could be expected to be substantial, while slightly less than those required to establish memorials. Frederick K. Upton chaired this special gift committee which had a three-week period to complete its solicitations with the help of forty of Concord's young business and professional men.

Ralph Avery led the charge during the highly visible public campaign. A claims manager for the Merchants Mutual Casualty Company, he was president of the Chamber of Commerce then. His 400-member group was organized in divisions by teams each having a captain, lieutenant, and six members. He was assisted by Mrs. Gardner Tilton and Natt Burbank. Mrs. Tilton, an active Red Cross worker, was also a Hospital Associates member and volunteer. Burbank was superintendent of the Union School District and a past member of the nursing school advisory committee.

Robert Potter, former legislator, alderman-at-large for Concord, and superintendent of buildings and grounds at St. Paul's School, headed the allied towns division covering thirty communities surrounding Concord.

As they began working, the *Concord Monitor* cranked up its publicity campaign even more, listing every worker's name, describing every meeting, urging all workers to attend each session to receive assignments and to turn in pledges. A thaw in the freezing weather was recorded on January 20. The ice breakup would aid in the achievement of 100 percent attendance at that evening's building fund meeting. The next day Langley praised the community unity which had brought 250 people to the meeting in the worst weather of the winter.

Daily newspaper articles were supplanted by small boxed items featuring a single idea. One illustrated "Wheels! Concord Hospital literally moves on them," recounting the various kinds of wheels involved in a patient's hospital stay from meal arrival on a heated cart to the stretcher on wheels and the rolling overbed table. Another box cartooned the routing of "busy little germs" by the five kinds of sulfa stocked in the hospital pharmacy.

Editorials written by Langley interpreted the trustees' intentions with regard to the communty's needs. Seldom has a campaign been so enthusiasti-

cally and so thoroughly supported by a news medium. By the opening day
of the public solicitation, over $700,000 of the one million dollars needed
had been subscribed.

The little boxes continued, one on the special faucets on the scrub sinks
used by surgeons who must scrub for ten minutes preceding an operation,
another on the lead-lined x-ray therapy room used to irradiate and shrink
a cancerous tumor.

More contributions were tallied, some with interesting sources such as
the $369 from the Concord Community War Gardens. The victory garden
movement had begun in Concord with two tracts of land made available
by former Mayor Charles J. Mckee and the late Joseph Walker. Each gar-
dener contributed approximately $2 a year toward the cost of plowing, har-
rowing, and the eventual restoration of the land to its original state. The
balance remaining in this fund after expenses were paid following the war
was the sum subscribed to the hospital fund.[3]

A week before the campaign was to end, James Langley wrote an editorial
warning the community that much remained to be done. The two existing
hospital plants must be sold and government funding obtained before construction could begin. He called the entire process a fifteen-year job.

*The first five-year phase was concerned with effecting consolidation of
Concord's general hospitals. That is past. That second phase has been concerned with building a new hospital. We are about in the middle of this
phase. But when Concord Hospital opens its doors there will still be a five-
year phase left-refinement of the hospital organization until we have the best
in medical care. Such organization does take time.[4]*

On February 14 with $989,538 in hand, campaign leaders decided to ex-
tend the drive another week at the request of volunteers who blamed the
bad traveling weather for their inability to solicit contributions in the out-
lying towns. Enthusiasm seemed undimmed at what was thought to be the
final reporting meeting. Several divisions announced that they had exceed-
ed their goals including the ones commanded by Alvin R. Hussey, James
Ross, and Mrs. Donald McIvor. Hussey's division led the men's teams and
Mrs. McIvor's the women's. The *Monitor* termed the closing meeting on
February 21 a victory celebration when volunteers gathered in Concord High
School's auditorium added $131,758 in new pledges to send the fund total
to $1,121,129, a 12 percent oversubscription.

Langley praised the nearly 1,000 volunteers with special mention of
memorial gifts committee members physicians Robert Graves and James
Jameson whose efforts brought in $130,000 from area doctors. Treasurer

Frank Sulloway paid tribute to the editor calling him the "prime mover" having raised over $200,000 himself.

Among the teams, the men came in first with 1,253 contributions totalling $40,068, although the women's teams had secured more contributions, 1,308 for a total of $35,836. Alvin Hussey's division was indeed, first with the top team captained by Lorne F. Lea, and Mrs. McIvor's division led the women volunteers with her ranking team captained by the tireless Margaret Emmons.

Looking over the dozens of articles and photographs devoted to the drive in the *Concord Monitor* reminds us that the era of such journalistic embrace of an essentially private cause has probably passed. Today, fund raisers automatically add production and mailing costs of the direct mail approach replacing or supporting the personal call.

Confident that it would be only a year or two before the new building's rise on Pleasant Street, the trustees turned their attention to the problems inherent in the operation of the two old hospitals. Standards for patient care were rising rapidly; Conant Faxon was eager to bring the new hospital organization up to the level demanded by the American College of Surgeons, while the school of nursing would aim toward standards developed by the National League for Nursing Education. Elizabeth Smith, RN had been hired to begin this task in September 1946 when the first class would enter the Concord Hospital School of Nursing. She left after one year.

New personnel were hired that year and the next to handle consolidated tasks. Dr. James Park was named pathologist; Mrs. Madeline Dane, admitting officer; Clifton Lord became pharmacist; and Frances Austin arrived to supervise housekeeping activities, and Cyril Kotrady the laundry. Dr. Robert Nydegger joined the surgical staff in 1946 and Angus Brooks, M.D. began the anesthesia department with his appointment to the staff in August 1947. Remembering that summer, Dr. Brooks, retired from the staff and now an active volunteer at Concord Hospital, said that he had no idea what to expect of the nurses who had been giving anesthesia when he arrived. When a patient called the department on the phone and requested that Dorothy Champigny put her to sleep, he met and formed a warm working relationship with the nurse who was to be a mainstay of his department for many years.[5]

Inasmuch as there were a multitude of issues to resolve surrounding the consolidation, it is surprising that most of them were settled between the parties involved. Evidently the question of the cap to be worn by graduate nurses in the hospital was not one of them because this issue was brought before the trustees. A motion to adopt the cap of the new Concord Hospital School of Nursing was defeated ten to eight. Sensitive to the loyalty students felt for their schools, trustees voted that students who had spent less than one and a half years in the Concord Hospital School would be permitted to choose between the hospital cap and that of the school they had entered before consolidation. Those who had spent the major portion of their training in the Concord Hospital School would wear the Concord cap. There may have been some doubt on the part of the public about the viability of this new school. The nursing school committee worried about the decrease in applications, enough to reduce the tuition in 1948 from $240 to $160. The next month six new students entered the school. The medical staff funded a $400 scholarship for one student to be used over the three-year course. An additional scholarship came from an anonymous donor.

Trustees were struggling with an inherited $100,000 deficit from the two earlier corporations while they dealt with the cost increases of the new institution. Because students were fewer following the war, graduate nurses were hired at higher salaries. An analysis of accounts receivable revealed a high proportion of unpaid bills from the outlying towns, a significant finding, for it prompted trustees to explore and later actively seek appropriations from the communities making up the hospital drawing area. For many years trustees visited yearly town meetings seeking support for the hospital on local warrants. One year, selectmen from the surrounding towns were invited to a dinner meeting to acquaint them with the work of the hospital. No direct solicitation was made that evening, but the idea was planted. Despite this kind of creativity (marketing today) on the part of trustees, few communities supported the hospital and those that did made only token appropriations. Yankee thrift did not extend to general support, though a town could be prevailed upon to extend charity to one of their own when they knew about a specific case. The hospital's benevolence was more visible within the city, for Concord was prompt in the payment of a yearly appropriation worked out between the city and its "citadel of health," the term coined by fund raisers.

Despite the signing of the Hill-Burton Act making federal funds available for construction, and despite the success of the fund drive, the building was no nearer construction in 1949 than at the time of the merger. It was discovered that an application for federal assistance could not even be initiated until final plans were drawn and the job ready to bid. James Langley, Willis Thompson, Jr., Pollie P. Thompson, Robert Potter, and Frank Sulloway were appointed the building committee, ready to take charge of the project in the event it became possible to build. Unrestricted endowment funds had been wiped out and more than $100,000 was owed banks. The

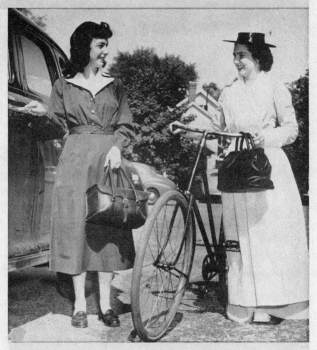

Incorporating **INDUSTRIAL NURSING**   **March 1950**

Trained Nurse
and Hospital Review
THE OLDEST NURSING JOURNAL IN AMERICA

•

COVER PHOTO
Two student nurses, Concord Hospital, portraying nursing of the District Nursing Association, Concord, N. H., fifty years ago and now. Madeline Finely, right, wearing uniform of 1899 and Pauline Boulay in the present uniform. See story on page 116)

The March 1950 Trained Nurse and Hospital Review *featured the District Nursing Association, fore-runner of the Concord Regional Visiting Nurse Association, now a part of the hospital's parent organization. Student Madeline Finley's name was spelled incorrectly here on the cover.*

community's enthusiasm for the hospital was waning as the cost of a stay in one of the old buildings rose alarmingly. Patients shortened their stays, driving costs even higher. Administrator Conant Faxon was discouraged to the point of requesting a change of officers to bring new ideas to trustee meetings. His plea was ignored, but help arrived in the form of a study by Bigelow, Kent, Willard & Company. Its report, issued on June 30, 1949, consisted of a number of findings and recommendations indicating that rates could be raised 20 percent to prevent further loss of capital and that the new hospital should be built within a year or two and be smaller than originally planned, 150 beds, expandable to 175. The rates were increased.

The medical staff prepared a major revision of its by-laws in 1949. A medical records committee was created to report delinquencies in records (physicians and dentists have procrastinated in this regard since records have been kept), and to propose cases for presentation at staff meetings. Members of the active staff would now be required to transfer to the consulting staff at age sixty-five. The term "service patient" (a patient who had no money to pay for hospitalization) was redefined as one "designated by the hospital as such" rather than one "admitted as such."

The administrator's relationship with his medical staff was deteriorating at the end of 1949. When Faxon was confronted by the executive committee he left, making it clear to all that he had been fired, though trustees had given him the opportunity to resign. The next day the hospital purchased back the house at 5 Grandview Avenue and the trustees began the search for a new administrator.

Robert Southwick, for five years the deputy superintendent of Washington, D.C.'s Gallinger Memorial Hospital, came to Concord on March 1, 1950, at a time when change was a daily occurrence. Plans for the new building were underway, the medical staff was attempting to conform with American College of Surgeons' recommendations and nursing education was making major strides. Standards for minimum qualifications of faculty were adopted, instruction and clinical experience in psychiatric nursing were made part of the nurse's education, and students in New Hampshire were now taking the new national licensing examination. Previously the examination had been administered by the state.

Alumnae of the school of nursing formalized their organization in 1950 by incorporating under the laws of New Hampshire. Their articles of incorporation in the name of The Alumnae Association of the Concord Hospital stated three objectives of the group. Section I reads: "For the mutual help and improvement of professional work and for the promotion of good fellowship among graduates of the school." Section II: "For the advancement

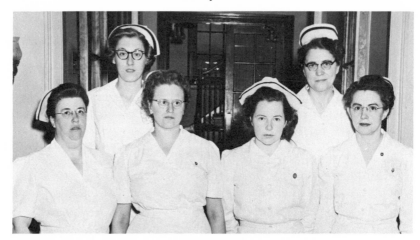

Head nurses pose at Margaret Pillsbury Hospital in the early fifties. Back row: Bertha McComish and Grace Stevens. Front row: Ruth Hagar, Helen Sargeant, Alice Maltais, and Doris Perkins.

of the interests of the Concord Hospital School of Nursing." Section III: "In cooperation with the New Hampshire State Nurses' Association, to work for the promotion of professional and educational advancement of nursing." Signing the articles of agreement were graduates Grace W. Stevens, Mary W. Kenney, Anne Shepard, Ruth H. Hagar, and Bessie L. Labor.

A visit from the executive secretary and director of the State Board of Nurse Examiners brought seven recommendations to the new school in 1950. The board of trustees was advised to reorganize the nursing school committee, the school should urge graduates to take post-graduate training. Job descriptions were recommended for faculty positions, and it was advised that nursing service and school budgets be separated. A second clinical affiliation should be obtained. The school was advised to stop taking February classes and to improve physical facilities.

All of these recommendations were adopted but not immediately. February classes were admitted until 1953 and trustees stubbornly refused to consider the separation of nursing service from the school for some years. Of course everyone concerned was eager to improve physical facilities. That would occur in two stages later on. One great advance probably not realized at the time was the engagement of Kathleen Clare, a New Hampshire native but recently of Richmond, Virginia, as educational director of the school. Nursing school faculty had come and gone. Kathleen Clare taught students and directed the school for more than thirty-three years, introducing

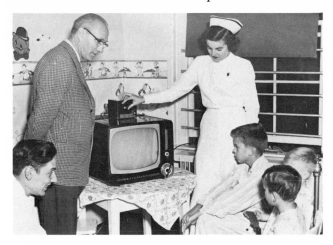

Dr. MacLean Gill, a pediatrician, observes as young patients gather, perhaps for Howdy Doody, when television came to the hospital in 1952.

advancements in nursing education, improving the quality of faculty and leaving a stamp of excellence recognized throughout the realm of diploma nursing programs.

Meanwhile, the trustees were engaged in their ongoing battle to cover the growing deficit. They voted to ask all three of the local banks to increase their loans to the hospital, the funds to be applied to accounts payable, vowing at the same time that it would be the last borrowing they would do.

In September 1950 Dr. Eugene McCarthy, president of the medical staff, called trustees' attention to the ominous news that fifteen New Hampshire doctors had been drafted, fortunately only one from Concord's staff. The Korean War had begun, another setback for the building plans, as federal funds were cut back, providing a total of $800,000 rather then the million dollars expected for construction purposes. Dr. Robert Rainie joined the staff that month at a time when the board was casting about for solutions to their money woes. Ranging from a proposal to close part of the hospital to an appeal to property taxpayers, their ideas reflected the degree of desperation the trustees felt. They did make a formal agreement with the Community Chest, forerunner of the United Way, which provided some funds for a few years.

The Hospital Associates, basking in the luxury of a large group of committed volunteers, initiated several of the projects in which they are engaged today. Mrs. Ross Mintz was chairman of the new Hospitality Shop which opened January 1, 1951, at the Pillsbury unit. The Associates began supervising the delivery of flowers to patients. Maternity patients at the Memorial unit were invited to purchase photos of their new babies taken soon after birth with a special camera located in the nursery.

A landmark advance for hospital employees occurred at the end of 1950 when the hospital elected to participate in the social security program, recently extended to non-profit organizations.

Students in the nursing school travelled to Columbus, Ohio, for two affiliations at midcentury. The medical and pediatric affiliation with Bellevue Hospital had been terminated when adequate housing for students could not be provided in New York City. A new alliance was forged with The Children's Hospital in Columbus, and when a clinical experience in infectious diseases (primarily tuberculosis) was needed, the closest institution that met the school's requirements was Benjamin Franklin Hospital, also in Columbus. Students endured a twenty-two-hour day coach ride on the train from Concord with box lunches packed by their classmates assigned to the diet kitchen. Psychiatric nursing was taught and experienced clinically at the New Hampshire Hospital here in Concord.

Two pages in the 1951 *Nutrix*, the student yearbook, were devoted to an impressive list of social functions students attended over their three-year course in those days. There were dances at New England College in Henniker and at Grenier Air Force Base in Manchester, a formal affair at St. Paul's School, and a spring dance at the Country Club sponsored by the medical staff. Parties were held at both units and the hospital family turned out in force for a summer picnic at Newfound Lake. One long-remembered Christmas gala at the Memorial unit featured a quartet of bogus Scandinavians whose hilarious renditions of "Yingle Bells" and "I Yust Go Nuts at Christmas" belied their everyday roles in white coats as anesthesiologist Angus Brooks, surgeons Robert Nydegger and Maurice Green and ear, nose and throat specialist Frank Perron. Encouraged by an enthusiastic reception a return engagement the following year found the four incognito again as hillbilly songsters mangling "Molasses" and "The Thing," which turned out to be Dr. McCarthy in a large box. History mercifully draws a blank on further appearances of this gang of four.

In December 1950 James Langley sat down at his *Monitor* desk and wrote a three-page letter to the hospital board stating firmly that he would not be a candidate for reelection at the March annual meeting. The letter was a summation of his years of activity on behalf of health care in New Hampshire and particularly of this work with Memorial Hospital and the merger. Obviously proud of his achievements he was also reluctant to give up entirely his involvement, offering to remain a trustee and member of the building committee which had not yet discharged its duty to see through the construction of the new building. Near the end of the letter he struck what was undoubtedly an uncharacteristic note for Langley, a note of wistful, even apologetic sadness as he acknowledged that he had not always been easy to get along with, increasingly so of late as he tried to accomplish too much. He allowed that his was the broad picture to paint, that it was best for others to fill in the details. It was a gracious letter from a man who described himself as "sometimes petulant, at times lazy, now and then dictatorial, always proud and seldom a gentleman."[6]

He was presented a citation for fifteen years of meritorious service to the combined hospitals on March 7, 1951, at the annual meeting which elected Concord businessman Roy Peaslee to the board presidency, but Langley remained a trustee long enough to lay the cornerstone of the new building in 1956.

New on the hospital scene then, the Red Cross blood bank was replacing individual hospital banks with a more efficient method of collecting and storing blood for future use. At first hearing the trustees voted against joining the Red Cross movement. At the following month's meeting organizers of the program, who needed participation by all of the state's large hospitals to make it work, made a presentation to the board, whereupon they voted to join.

The American College of Surgeons gave the hospital a 90 percent rating in 1951 with reservations concerning the physical plant. Horace S. Blood, son of the former governor joined the staff early in the year, a few months before the death of Dr. Carleton Metcalf, a longtime staff member who had contributed many advances to the practice of medicine at Margaret Pillsbury Hospital.

The subject of the forty-hour work week contributed to the length of board meetings in 1952 as that trend was hotly debated by trustees. Our thrifty New England businessmen were reluctant to join the move although they did give Superintendent of Nurses Winifred Hodgkins permission to experiment with the plan as long as costs would not be increased and providing it could be extended to all hospital departments. According to the records, trustees were wary of the idea, but the administrator assured them that all Boston hospitals had begun observing the forty-hour work week and it would have to be faced here sooner or later. The question was referred to the executive committee for a decision. The trial period was not popular with nurses who were already the lowest paid of any in the state according to an

American Hospital Association survey. In 1952 nurses here started at $175 per month compared with the New England average of $209 and the national average of $224. A higher rate scale was prepared but not voted on at the meeting at which it was proposed. Reluctance to grant pay increases was symptomatic of the general feeling of discouragement among the trustees. They were continually at work on schemes to save money. Tuition at the nursing school was brought back up from $160 to $299 while a study was underway to determine the cost of operating the school. Miss Hodgkins was complimented on keeping her payroll low. The study, one of many since its 19th century beginnings proved, as past surveys had, that the school's operation kept the hospital deficit down by furnishing student nurses to care for patients. The hospital's increased costs were partly the result of higher wages of graduate nurses taking the place of private duty nurses, and replacing some student duty. Students now spent more time in classes and less on the floors. Samuel Richmond of St. Paul's School assisted the committee in determining whether the school was overstaffed. They concluded that the pupil load per instructor was reasonable. While the school was clearly an expense to the hospital, the cost of replacing care given by students would be greater than the costs they were incurring. It was noted in the report that the physical setup of the two hospitals made cuts in nursing personnel impossible.

The committee's recommendation to continue the school did not include a vote for salary increases. Franklin Hollis, the attorney who headed the committee (his mother Amoret Hollis had headed it for twenty years), was of the opinion that nursing care must be cut, but was aware that some nurses might be lost including the school's new educational director. They asked the administrator to be prepared at the next meeting with a list of nursing services the hospital could cut. In the meantime they would try to sell the Grandview Avenue house to create a capital asset for building purposes. Unpaid pledges from the fund drive were to be solicited. The South Street Downing building of the Memorial unit was now in use as a treatment ward for alcoholic patients, operated by the state but staffed by Concord Hospital which derived revenue from those patients. Donation Day was still providing a little cash, about $1,000 and provisions in the form of jellies and jams (125 jars in 1952), cereals, sugar, molasses, chickens, acorn squash, and four table cloths. One trustee reported the receipt of three bushels of potatoes solicited a month earlier in Suncook and recently received "through patience and diplomacy." Fred Davis, who lived next door to the new hospital property gave a strip of land adjoining the building site making it possible to design an approach to the west side of the building.

In the early fifties Concord Hospital and most of its staff physicians attracted the kind of notoriety ordinarily shunned by the medical profession.

At midcentury great advances had been made toward conquering a few of the killer diseases of the period. Pneumonia was no longer feared and much had been accomplished to increase the life span of the diabetic. Cancer research was in its infancy, however, leaving the door open to quackery and the dubious remedies that had not yet been tested for effectiveness. A Massachusetts practitioner, Dr. Robert E. Lincoln of Medford, professed to have what he called a cure-all that could benefit cancer, tuberculosis, blindness, and other unrelated ailments. Giving credence to the cure-all locally, Charles W. Tobey, Jr., son of United States Senator Tobey, claimed to have been cured of lung cancer at the Lincoln Institute.[7]

The cure-all, bacteriophages alpha and beta created from two strains of staphylococcus, was administered (through inhalation) at the Lincoln Institute and by "fellows" of this institution, physicians who had been trained there. The remedy had not been subjected to the usual scientific testing given drugs before releasing them for general use and Dr. Lincoln was on no hospital staff, nor was he associated with any medical school where such testing might have been carried out.

Late in 1951 James Langley wrote an editorial debunking the treatment and its practitioners, referring obliquely to its use by a Concord physician. During 1952 a suit was filed in Merrimack County Superior Court bringing the full story to the public.[8]

Four patients who had been treated with the cure-all by Dr. Thomas Matthews were suing Concord Hospital and as many of its medical staff as were present at a staff meeting at which Matthews was allegedly threatened with dismissal if he continued to administer the Lincoln treatment. One patient who had been diagnosed with cancer had made arrangements for his funeral when he began treatment with Dr. Matthews, whereupon his condition steadily improved. A housewife with eczema began treatment and was gradually improving. The third patient was a victim of multiple sclerosis (defined by the *Monitor* as "creeping paralysis"), and the fourth had ulcerative colitis. All four claimed the need to continue the treatment in Concord, calling it a hardship to make the trip to Medford to receive the bacteriophages. The four were represented by none other than Charles Tobey, Jr. Hospital staff members were represented by Concord's leading attorneys: Frederick K. Upton of Upton, Sanders and Upton; Irving Soden of Sulloway, Jones, Piper, Hollis and Godfrey; Atlee Zellers and Mayland H. Morse, Jr., of Morse, Hall and Morse. Charles Toll of Orr and Reno represented the hospital.[9]

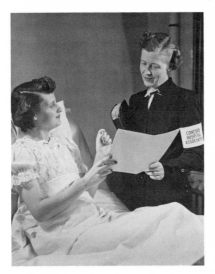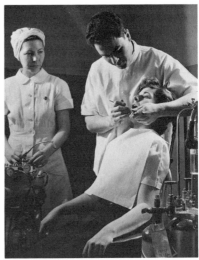

After much delay a two-day trial was finally convened in early May 1953. A few physicians petitioned to be eliminated as defendants by virtue of not being present when the alleged offense had occurred. Arguments for dismissal of the complaint presented by the defendants' counsel centered on the fact that the suit asked the hospital and doctors to stop doing things which they were not authorized to do anyway, such as prevent Dr. Matthews from practicing medicine, barring him from the hospital staff, and keeping him from administering the Lincoln treatment to his patients. Only the State Board of Registration could stop him from practicing and the physicians could not bar him from their staff; only the hospital as an institution could do so.[10]

The newspaper accounts of the hearing are exhaustive and as exciting as one is likely to read when such an event features most of the city's best known physicians testifying against one of their own, virtually all of the legal talent in town, the son of a U.S. senator, and a doctor of questionable reputation. "L.A. Law" meets "St. Elsewhere" on Main Street.

Attorney Tobey rested his case against the hospital and dismissals were eventually granted to seven of the original thirty-four physicians named in the suit. Counsel for the remaining twenty-seven rested their case and were given a few days to file briefs on behalf of their clients. Judge Harold Westcott dismissed charges against the group stating that they had acted in good faith in advising, not ordering Matthews to discontinue use of the treatment, their conduct was fair and reasonable and the means were proper under all

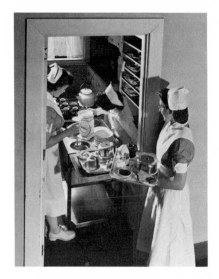

The publicity photos shown on these and the following page were taken for the completion fund drive in the mid-fifties. At far left Helen Mintz, who was heavily involved in the Concord Hospital Associates, shows a new mother a picture of her baby. Dr. Wendell Fitts is shown at work in the center photo, and at right, student nurses prepare patient trays in the diet kitchen.

of the circumstances. Dr. Matthews had testfied that he would no longer administer the Lincoln treatment no matter what the outcome of the trial. Dr. Lincoln was censured in a twenty-seven page report of the Massachusetts Medical Society which challenged the efficacy of the treatment and asked him to resign from the society. The society's investigating committee reported that the senator's son underwent surgery and received x-ray treatment before he was treated by Dr. Lincoln, destroying any credibility for the treatment. The *New England Journal of Medicine* denounced the treatment and accused Senator Tobey of using the *Congressional Record* to promote its use.[11]

On the heels of the Lincoln affair came a letter to the hospital from the New Hampshire Department of Health which made further delay in construction untenable. It stated rather succinctly that the Concord Hospital must begin construction of its new building not later than the spring of 1953 or federal funds in the amount of one million dollars would be reallocated to one or both of the other projects planned in New Hampshire (Hanover and Dover). The letter, dated June 4, asked for a project application to present to the Hospital Advisory Council's June 20 meeting. While the board must have been perturbed at the speed with which they would be required to act, act they did.

By June 9 executive and building commitees had met and architects had estimated costs of a revised plan bringing the project's cost down to

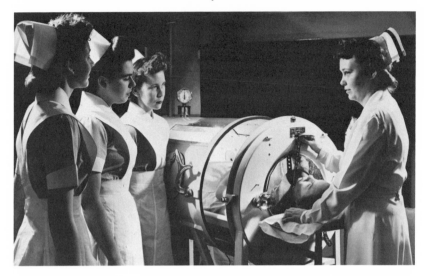

Polio was a real threat in the 1950s and many patients endured long periods in an iron lung, here demonstrated to an attentive class.

$3,200,000 by eliminating the nurses' home. The original application for Hill-Burton funds, an announcement of intention to build, had already been filed. The revised building plans would constitute part II of the application, and trustees voted to submit that section to the Hospital Advisory Council.

The nursing school was, at that time, operating under a temporary accreditation of the National League for Nursing, one of seven of New Hampshire's thirteen schools to be so accredited during the first evaluations by the organization. Director Hodgkins, Kathleen Clare, and Assistant Director of Nursing Claire O'Neil requested permission to attend the national meeting of the NLN in Boston. Administrator Southwick recommended that the request be denied in the light of a state effort to standardize nursing education which should be supported instead.

In June Winifred Hodgkins who had directed both nursing service and the school resigned, and the administrator saw an opportunity to reorganize the school under a director, and to hire a separate director for the nursing service. Inquiries revealed disapproval of that plan within the state board of nursing, so once more a single individual was sought to fill both positions. It must have been welcome news to read in the paper that a Memorial Hospital graduate, Lieutenant Mildred Rush, of Pembroke, would be receiving an award in Washington from the Women's National Press Club as their "woman of the year." Rush had taken a year's post-graduate work in anesthesia at the Massachusetts General Hospital and had become a member of that hospital's staff of nurse anesthetists. She entered the Army Nurse Corps in 1950 and after an assignment at Brooke Army Hospital, Fort Sam Houston, Texas, was assigned to a mobile Army surgical hospital (MASH) in Korea, serving fifteen months there, longer than the usual tour of duty. She would accept the award on behalf of all nurses serving in Korea who were compositely "woman of the year."

Trustees had asked the help of Will, Folsum and Smith to mount a fund drive to augment building funds. The executive committee asked Dudley Orr to chair that drive. Bids were opened prior to the June trustees meeting at which it was announced that the Davison Construction Company of Manchester had submitted the lowest bid.

The campaign to complete the financing of the new structure opened in September 1953 with a dinner at the Eagle Hotel where Dudley Orr gave board President Roy Peaslee the opportunity to answer questions about the delay. Citing the Korean war as the reason Hill-Burton funds had been cut and inflation for the increase in the cost of the building, he hastened to assure listeners that monies from the original fund drive were earning interest, much of it in government bonds. James Langley described the existing hospital buildings as the oldest in the state with the wooden buildings badly termite-infested, plumbing, heating, and wiring in poor condition. The new hospital would solve all of these problems adding services for which no space existed now such as central sterile supply, emergency operating rooms, and outpatient services. No longer would patients be placed on long waiting lists for elective surgery. Langley cannily avoided discussion concerning the school of nursing stating that the new building "will allow for economical expansion of services as needed, the addition of a new school of nursing for which plans have already been drawn . . . . "

Even as construction began, the trustees grappled with the problem of the nursing school. Money was so tight that it was decided to close the Memorial unit's nurses' residence, moving students into the Pillsbury residence, saving $1,000. They were forced to scrap a 1940 Chevrolet truck used to transport laundry between units and they were dickering with the fund raisers on the costs of the campaign while worrying about the construction costs they were about to incur.

In the midst of this unpleasantness Robert Southwick resigned. Trustees lost no time in locating a replacement bringing Norman R. Brown from Claremont within a month.

Brown, now retired and living in Rye, New Hampshire, remembers the low ebb at which he found both hospital and nursing school in May, 1955.

"There were a few footings in the ground for the new building and no money to pay for them." The dietition became upset one day when the local supplier refused to leave any eggs until his bill was paid. Even the phone company threatened to cut service to the hospital when its bill became long overdue. Brown recalled visiting the top floor ward at the Pillsbury building and wondering why there were squares and circles painted on the floor. The head nurse explained that these were the locations for basins to be placed under leaks in the old slate roof.[12]

Salaries were so low that the director's position for nursing service and the school went unfilled. Morale was very low at the school where students made do with the old pest house as their classroom, it being the only space large enough for student assembly. When the Memorial unit students moved into Pillsbury's residence a little more cohesiveness was achieved at the cost of crowding.

No applicants had appeared for the directorship, so Kathleen Clare and Claire O'Neil, who were sharing the work, went to the administrator and asked to assume formally the positions of school director and director of nursing service. This was a radical change and Brown remembers that he was at first dubious. "But," he said, "both of these women were capable and knew what they were doing. If anyone but Clare and O'Neil had asked, I probably would not have agreed to the plan." He added that their success in dividing the job set the tone for a number of schools that attempted the same change later.

Brown began to make many such changes in the hospital's administration with the help of Ella Siegler, who had been at the hospital for some years as secretary to the director and was now his administrative assistant. Some changes came about through recommendations of the new Joint Commission on the Accreditation of Hospitals which inspected the hospital for the first time in June 1954.

The first major move was to reduce the nursing staff from 132 to 111 at the same time granting the first third of a $15 a month pay raise. He recommended extensive rate changes and a reduction in benefits of the hospital's Blue Cross program in which the institution would pay one half of the employee's basic premium. He also attacked the problem of the hospital's older employees. At the end of 1953 some twenty-two employees were over the age of seventy, many of them working in the dietary department. A training program was planned to introduce employees to the advanced techniques to be used in the new building. Those who could not adapt would be retired.

In 1954, the year that Webster Soule was appointed to the staff in internal medicine, the essential fairness of the trustees was made manifest in their

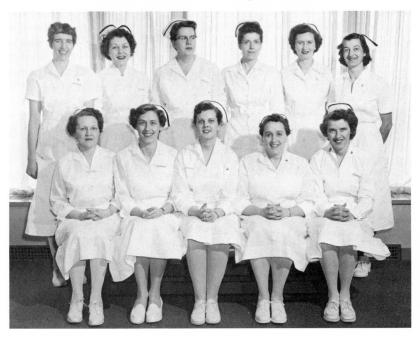

Nursing supervisors at Concord Hospital, about 1956. Back row: Ona Clouette, (unidentified), Eunice Newhall, Lois Carter, Mary Watterson, Rita Perry. First row: Anna Estabrook, Bertha McComish, Eveleana Gifford, Carrie Jenovese, Margaret Wallace.

opposition to an effort on the part of the medical staff to control the kind and number of new practitioners coming into the community. Led by attorneys Dudley Orr and Frank Sulloway, the trustees went on record as opposed to any effort by the staff to regulate their own incomes by opposing competition from new practitioners. If qualified, such applicants should be admitted to the staff. Time has proven the soundness of this attitude which prevails today.

By March 1955 it had been decided that the school of nursing should occupy temporary quarters encompassing the four wings of the new building's fifth floor. The State Board of Nursing gave its approval to this plan with the stipulation that facilities meeting all of their requirements must be provided by 1961. The administrator's approval was added to that of trustees Dudley Orr and Margaret Emmons. Banks expressed willingness to loan money on the commitment of the hospital's endowment funds, and the architects waived any claim to additional fees for more construction.

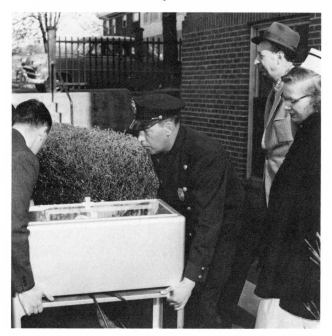

*Moving day, May, 1956. Administrator Norman Brown, at right, watches
as police transfer a tiny patient in an incubator to a waiting ambulance for
the ride from Spring Street to 250 Pleasant Street.*

Accounts payable were down from $63,000 to $16,000 in just one year, and plans to open the new hospital with a fanfare (literally so, for the musician's union planned to donate a ten-piece band for the occasion), were underway. At the end of 1955 when internist John Argue of Pittsfield and dentist Richard Lassonde joined medical and dental staffs, the outlook for Concord Hospital had brightened considerably. A sizable grant from the Ford Foundation became available for construction purposes and agreement had been reached with the state for the sale of the Memorial unit for $125,000. The community was rallying round the move to the new building as the trustees planned dedication ceremonies for spring when the weather would presumably be cooperative.

10

Growth and the End of an Era

ary Watterson was on duty one stormy evening in the spring of 1956 at the old Margaret Pillsbury Hospital. She recalled the evening for the hospital's employee publication *Life Lines* thirty-three years later at the time of her retirement. Her unit included a converted sunporch which leaked. When a gust of wind blew the door open in walked a wet cat that began to groom itself. "Laughing at this unauthorized guest, a visitor remarked, 'Well, I guess we do need a new hospital.'"[1]

The dedication ceremony for the new building was presided over on April 14, 1956, by Douglas N. Everett, then president of the board of trustees, and as in earlier dedications, the governor, this time Lane Dwinell, and Mayor Howe Anderson were present to lend an official air to the proceedings. The major speaker was Richard Viguers of the New England Hospital Assembly, but the real star of the occasion as all present must have realized was James Langley, who laid the cornerstone, cementing in records of the merger and fund drive and a student yearbook. It was the year Langley received an honorary doctor of laws degree from the University of New Hampshire and the year before his appointment by President Eisenhower as ambassador to Pakistan, a post he would hold for two years before returning to Concord and the *Concord Monitor*.

The small pamphlet given to those who attended the ceremony and toured the new building provides us the statistics for 1955: Admissions totalled 5,045, births 901. Hopkinton was the area town with the largest number of admissions, 203. The number of operations that year was 3,806. Hospital

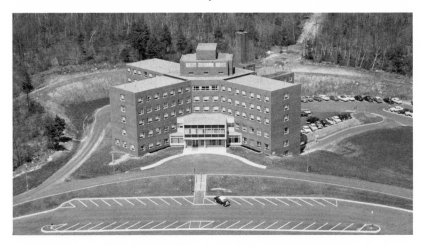

The new Concord Hospital at 250 Pleasant Street shortly before its opening in 1956.

employees and nurses numbered 225, while there were 69 student nurses and 74 members of the medical, dental, and surgical staffs.[2]

Mary Watterson remembered in her *Life Lines* interview that construction was not completely finished two weeks after the dedication when the hospital opened. The nursing units lacked water and buckets had to be hauled from the kitchen. The board minutes record a promise from St. Paul's School to provide meals on the day of the move and some recall that trucks were donated by several firms to move equipment and supplies. Students moved to their new fifth floor quarters on May 14, Memorial patients on May 15 and Pillsbury patients the next day.

Not everything was new and shiny. The administrator resourcefully had some of the old furniture redone and metal was refinished at New Hampshire Hospital's workshop. A long conference table was acquired at half-price when it was rejected as not meeting the requirements of the Monday Review Club. Medical records prior to 1930 were destroyed rather than moved.

Amos Mansur was awarded the contract to demolish the main Pillsbury building, now an empty hulk and prey to vandalism. A group of physicians was formed to purchase its annex bringing into the world the group practice known as the Concord Clinic. The McKerley family purchased its nurses' residence which became McKerley's nursing home.

The happiest residents of the new hospital were the students and faculty of the school of nursing ensconced on the fifth floor in what Norman Brown termed not in the least luxurious quarters. They were, however, all in one location, needing only to take the elevator to enter the clinical area. What a change from the recent past when one might live on South Street and have to walk to South Main Street for a class and back to South Spring Street to go on duty on a maternity ward.

Even as a new class was settling in, the State Board of Nursing asked for a clarification of what must be included in temporary housing for students. Franklin Hollis was angry and lost no time in replying to the Board expressing surprise at this request because the Board had already approved the housing arrangements. He was able to settle the question diplomatically without further fuss.

The *Nutrix* for 1956 carried several pictures of the various places the students had called home: the old Memorial residence, Pillsbury's nurses' home, and the new hospital, raw and unlandscaped on the Pleasant Street hill. The yearbook pictures too, a new pediatric affiliation at the Boston Children's Medical Center where the girls claimed the main attraction was Harvard Medical School, seen from a window.

There were comings and goings in 1956 and 1957. Dr. Donald McIvor was honored with the dedication of the students' yearbook as he retired in June 1956 after thirty-seven years on the staff. Grace Stevens retired the next year. She had been at the hospital as a head nurse nearly all of the thirty-four years since her graduation from Margaret Pillsbury's training school. A member of the first nursing school advisory committee after the merger, she continued to serve on that committee for several years after her retirement and was long active in alumni affairs. Margaret Emmons also retired from that committee, which she had served as a trustee member for years, shortly before her death.

Dr. Munro Proctor arrived to begin the practice of internal medicine and later, cardiology in 1957, and it was the year in which Norman Brown suggested that the hospital hire a director of volunteers as nearly all hospitals of 200 beds or more had one. The Associates agreed to this idea offering to provide $1,000 of her salary. They sought an experienced social worker who might aid persons leaving the hospital as well as locate outside sources of volunteer help. Mrs. Dorothy Smith became the first volunteer director, but it is Ruth Hungerford whom many remember as a longtime director of volunteers.

Studies were underway again on the cost of operating the school. One survey indicated that while a cash saving of $86,000 would result if the school were closed, it would cost from $80,000 to $90,000 to staff the hospital. It was reported that the cost then of operating the school would not be materi-

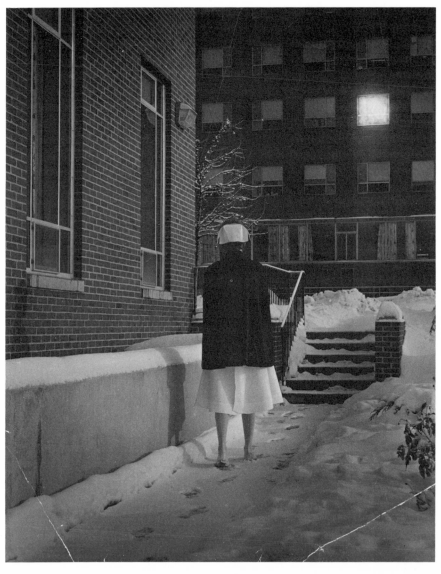

A student begins the evening shift with a short walk through the snow to the hospital. A less picturesque route would have taken her through the basement tunnel connecting the buildings.

ally increased with the addition of a separate nurses' home and an increase in revenue would accrue from the additional space gained for patients on the fifth floor. At that time 41 percent of the nursing staff were the hospital's own graduates. To replace student nurses would require 27 registered nurses, 7 practical nurses and 2 aides. With only 54 nurses on the local registry, it would be difficult to staff the hospital without recruiting outside the Concord area. Possible changes in the education of nurses were discussed, but all agreed that no matter what degrees might be sought by nurses they would still be required to have at least two years of clinical training which could only be accomplished in hospitals, therefore, a nurses' home would be needed in any case.

The trustees at this executive committee session were putting themselves through an exercise, statistical, rhetorical, in order to decide what kind of structure might meet the needs of the hospital. It was reported that Keene State College had recently built a dormitory for $220,000, St. Paul's School for $275,000. The administrator had recently made a preliminary "notice of intent to construct" which requested some $1,500,000 in federal aid for a nurses' home.

As one can guess, the nursing school committee was proposing a nurses' home consisting solely of living space at that juncture.

The school was then in the midst of the evaluation process seeking full accreditation from the National League for Nursing for the first time. Franklin Hollis noted at a board meeting that in six years only 311 of the 955 schools in the United States had been accredited, hinting that the demands on schools were great and that our school might not receive accreditation. (Provisional accreditation was granted in January 1958.)

Recognizing that the hospital's fifth floor quarters would be somewhat confining for a group of healthy young women, Drs. Ellsworth Tracy and Ross Mintz proposed to the medical staff that a small cottage be built in the woods behind the hospital. They thought a $4,000 to $5,000 expenditure might provide a lodge with fireplace, lights, and water (perhaps the cost was underestimated for Dr. Jameson later gave the money to install plumbing). To the staff contribution would be added that year's proceeds from Donation Day. By October the building was ready and the name, chosen in a contest, became aptly The Chatterbox. It served students for some years as an ideal place to blow off steam after a long day's work. Later on, unhappily, students were forbidden to use the Chatterbox after dark. There were no security personnel available to accompany them.

In 1959, Douglas Everett, who had guided the hospital through the com-

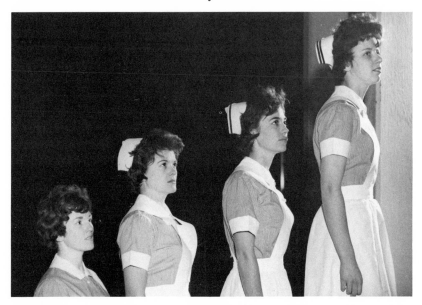

The school catalog titled this photo "stepping-stones to success." It portrays the stages of progress through the program from the freshman in the first three months of school to the second stage after receiving cap and apron bib. The second-year student wears one stripe on the cap border, the senior, two.

pletion fund drive and building process retired as president of the board. Everett, who headed a local insurance and real estate agency, had won fame in his Dartmouth student days as a member of the silver medallist ice hockey team in the 1932 Olympic games. As a trustee he contributed generously his knowledge of the insurance industry to the board's deliberations.

Ralph Avery took the hospital into the sixties, overseeing the next construction project, a school of nursing building. By May 1959, the building committee and administrator had decided to construct a combination classroom building and residence for student nurses, although there were indications that the future of nursing was in for a good deal of educational upheaval.

In that year, Paul Lena, a resident physician at Mary Hitchcock Hospital in Hanover agreed to a locum tenens period in Concord covering for Dr. J. Dunbar Shields, and Dr. Bernard A. Gouchoe was elected to the hospital's courtesy staff.

The impetus for building the school came not only from the State Board of Nursing, but from the need for more beds in the hospital. The trustees were reassured by Franklin Hollis that there would be in the next few years a "staggering potential demand for nurses." He reviewed with the board the work of the Spaulding Council on Nursing Education whose studies suggested that although college courses might eventually become part of the training, no possibility existed then of abandoning hospital schools.

January 1960 brought full National League for Nursing accreditation to the school, one of five of the state's eleven schools to be so accredited. The board of trustees voted a resolution of congratulation to Kathleen Clare and her faculty for this accomplishment, a source of encouragement to fund raising and planning for the new building.

Koehler and Isaak, Inc. had submitted plans to the building committee, but James Langley favored revising the original drawings of Shepley, Bulfinch, Richardson and Abbott. Negotiations proceeded with both architectural firms while Will, Folsum and Smith recommended an $800,000 goal for the fund drive after canvassing a few large givers. Solicitation began on September 14, 1960. In the meantime, both of the architects were successful. Koehler and Isaak would design the school, and Shepley, Bulfinch, Richardson and Abbott was to submit plans for the fifth floor conversion to patient units. Optimistically, the Hospital Associates pledged $12,000 to the building fund in memory of the recently deceased Helen Mintz, first chairman of their thriving Hospitality Shop.

The staff was enlarged by three in the summer of 1960 when Drs. Thomas Ferraro, a urologist; Charles L. Ward, internist; and general practitioner Harold Conrad of Pittsfield were appointed to the courtesy staff.

Franklin Hollis in his role as chairman of the nursing school committee was the ideal choice to chair the fund-raising campaign in which he was aided by I. Reed Gourley with initial gifts and Edward Sanel, corporate gifts. The public solicitation effort would be managed by attorney Eugene Struckoff. Hill-Burton funds were to be available in the amount of $170,000, but Portsmouth Hospital had failed in its attempt to qualify for federal funds freeing an additional $30,000 for Concord's use. Davison Construction, Inc. was again the low bidder and they projected a completion date of April, 1962.

These were the years of "duck and cover" when nuclear disaster occupied everyone's spare thoughts to some extent, so, inevitably, preparation was made by the public sector to shelter and feed those who might be caught in a nuclear attack on New England. Back in 1957 the New Hampshire Hospital Association had sponsored a state-wide fire safety institute during which trained volunteers taught patient evacuation techniques and emergency fire fighting. Several of Concord Hospital's nursing staff were active

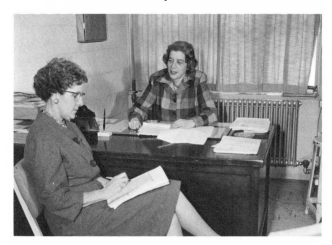

*Kathleen Clare (Yeaple) dictates to secretary Maybelle Brockway
in the temporary quarters of the nursing school on the hospital's
fourth and fifth floors.*

in the planning and operation of these sessions travelling across the state
to teach other hospital personnel. In 1961 Dr. Homer Lawrence, then medical staff president, reported that a disaster drill to be held in November
would enlist the aid of local Civil Defense officials with respect to protec-
tion against nuclear fallout.

The ultimate drill came in 1964 when a group of eighteen men and wom-
en, including Director of Nursing Eileen Wolseley, Kathleen Clare of the
school of nursing, Eunice Newhall, administrative supervisor of nursing
service, and purchasing agent Richard Johnson endured thirty-eight hours
of confinement in the underground shelter at the New Hampshire Savings
Bank. Part of a training course in shelter management, the group lived under survival conditions, their only food a daily ration of three special 100-
calorie biscuits developed by Civil Defense and six ounces of water with each
meal. Realistic messages on the state of the city and nation during an actu-
al disaster were communicated to the group by phone as they practiced ad-
justments to living in confined quarters and learned to read radiological
monitoring equipment. According to the *Monitor* article describing the drill,
the participants also learned a lot more about each other than they wanted
to know. One man commented that he would no longer believe that only
men snored.

The fund drive was successful beyond expectation bringing in about

$5,000 more than the building's expected cost of $920,000. Contributions from the large givers such as banks, the Hospital Associates, the nursing school alumnae, large corporations and the service clubs accounted for the first $100,000. Some 400 volunteers from Concord and the surrounding towns raised the rest in a public campaign. A glossy brochure offered memorial opportunities and featured on its cover Pamela Smith, a second year nursing student from Plymouth, posed with the traditional Florence Nightingale lamp. She was introduced to the more than 300 volunteers who attended an opening dinner at Rundlett Jr. High School. Pamela, serving as the symbol of the hospital and its service to the community, appeared almost daily in newspaper photos of checks being presented, pledge cards turned in and team captains reporting subscriptions.

Construction of the building was completed on time and dedicated on May 12, 1962, during American Hospital Week with James Langley again cementing in the cornerstone.[3] The hospital had purchased a silverplated tea service which was used for the first time during these festivities.

At the time of the dedication, the school received a good deal of publicity. It is possible that the *Monitor's* readers learned for the first time just how the school functioned and under what authority. The article printed in the May tenth issue described the school in detail with particular reference to the chain of command from the director to the administrator to the board of trustees through the nursing school committee. In 1962 Kathleen Clare was assisted by eight fulltime faculty members, a student health nurse, two science instructors, two housemothers and two secretaries. Members of the hospital's medical staff were still providing lectures and clinical instruction in the hospital. Nursing supervisors, head nurses, and hospital department heads also participated in the educational program which that year taught seventy-two students from Maine, New Hampshire, Vermont, Massachusetts, and Rhode Island.

The new building had, in addition to forty-seven dormitory rooms, two housemother's suites with bedroom, bath, and living room, six offices for faculty and administration, two classrooms, a science laboratory, a nursing arts classroom with eight practice beds, three conference rooms, a library, living room, recreation room, laundry, and an auditorium.

Now that the students were relocated in their new quarters the hospital turned its attention to the renovation of the fifth floor in order to add fifty-eight adult beds.

Benjamin Potter joined the courtesy staff in April 1962 to practice obstetrics and gynecology. Although new physicians were coming to Concord

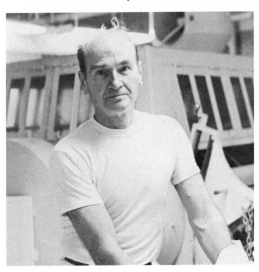

*Cyril "Cy" Kotrady in the laundry he operated for many
years at Pillsbury and Concord Hospitals before retirement.
Cy's spotless white shirt and trousers were emblematic of
the pride he took in the operation of this vital
hospital service.*

at a satisfying rate, hospitals were beginning to feel an acute shortage of
nurses. All kinds of ideas were entertained to alleviate the strain on patient
units. High school girls were being trained as aides with the hope that some
would choose nursing as a career. There was the added burden of the fifty-
eight new beds, so although they were not enthusiastic about the idea, a
selective care wing was opened for patients whose needs were less than acute.
Operating with more aides than nurses, the wing freed eighteen beds elsewhere in the hospital.

As problems at New Hampshire Hospital created a consolidation in nursing care there, Dorothy Breene, director of nursing, appealed to Concord
Hospital's school to accept students for affiliation in medical-surgical, pediatric, and operating room nursing. Not wishing to compromise its own
educational program, the school drew up a list of fourteen conditions upon
which the students would be accepted. These conditions were agreeable to
New Hampshire Hospital and the students arrived, to remain in affiliation
until that school closed in 1983. Later on when the associate degree program
at the New Hampshire Technical Institute was established, its students be-

gan a clinical affiliation with Concord Hospital which continues today.

Trustees took the time in 1963 to familiarize themselves with their growing hospital by attending a dinner in the cafeteria with department heads
who spoke about their work. Dr. Maurice Green was president of the medical staff, Ella Siegler represented administration, Kathleen Clare the nursing school, Esther Holt medical records, Irving Everson the business office,
Cyril Kotrady, the laundry, Mrs. Low, housekeeping. Dr. Winifred Sanborn
Mullins represented anesthesiology, Dr. James Park, pathology, Raymond
Reed, the pharmacy. Everett Thurston headed the maintenance department,
Dr. Frederick Waldron, radiology, and Eileen Wolseley, nursing service.

The Associates began a program in 1963 that has served as an effective
recruitment of nurses for many years. They voted a $500 donation to fund
two scholarships to the school of nursing. These awards were to be considered loans unless the recipients agreed to work at the hospital for one year
following graduation. The medical staff liked this idea so much that they
voted to increase their two scholarships to four on the same conditions. That
year Donation Day funds were earmarked for scholarship purposes and Dr.
and Mrs. Jameson donated $10,000, the income from which was to be spent
on scholarships for unmarried students.

The hospital opened a school for medical technologists that year similar
to the one they had begun for x-ray technologists eight years earlier. These
schools were in operation until no longer needed in the early seventies when
the New Hampshire Technical Institute developed programs to fill the needs
of the state's hospitals, physicians, and laboratories.

Franklin Hollis gave up his chairmanship of the nursing school committee in 1962 to devote more of his volunteer time to a modernization of the
hospital's financial organization, specifically the establishment of a common trust fund. Legislation had been passed in New Hampshire in 1959 al-
lowing trust funds held by nonprofit corporations to be grouped in this man-
ner, but the process of reading and analyzing each will and obtaining legal
opinions on the pertinent restrictions of some forty-five individual funds
was arduous and time-consuming. The committee, consisting of Hollis, his
son-in-law, banker David L. Stark, and Francis Southworth was ready in
February 1965 to recommend formation of a common trust fund to absorb
all but one or two funds such as the Jameson surgical instrument fund. The
common fund would be invested for the benefit of the hospital under the
terms of the resolution dated October 18, 1965, by the investment committee of the trustees. Bookkeeping would be greatly simplified as would the
investment process.

With the completion of the school building and renovation of the fifth

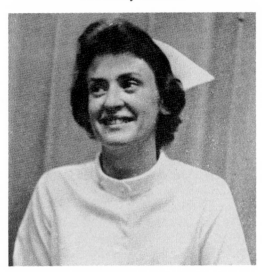

Elaine Manville (Hoyt) in 1964 when she taught medical-surgical nursing. She became director of the school of nursing in 1984.

floor, the trustees were able to pay off outstanding mortgages and announce that the hospital was debt free. Norman Brown was largely responsible for the first black ink seen at Concord Hospital, but he was not one to rest on his laurels, however honorably earned. There was an acute shortage of nurses and much to be done to attract new ones and to re-attract inactive ones. There was concern too, that New Hampshire hospitals might have to write off over $2 million dollars in the next three years because the legislature had not budgeted adequate reimbursement for the state's welfare patients. A nationwide trend was beginning to bring large numbers of patients into emergency rooms causing a strain on these facilities, and salaries throughout the hospital must be raised.

Staff nurse salaries were increased to $80 to $90 per week in 1965 with the base weekly pay for employees to become $50. Room rates were raised to pay for the increases.

The Medicare bill was signed by President Lyndon Johnson in 1965, and Concord Hospital received approval to begin accepting Medicare patients on July 1, 1966. This "great society" program, to be administered on the east and west coasts by Blue Cross-Blue Shield, was the first thread of the web of government intervention in health care pulled tighter and tighter every year since.

At the time in June when Robert O. Wilson, D.D.S., an oral surgeon, was appointed to the courtesy dental staff, Norman Brown was describing to trustees the preparations the hospital had made for Motorcycle Weekend, a new yearly event in Concord when hundreds of cycles roared through the city on their way to Loudon's Bryar Motorsport Park. Most physicians expected to be on call that weekend as the hospital braced for an influx of accidents. There were accidents, but not more than could be managed easily by the emergency room, and they have decreased in each succeeding year the event has been held.

In their own building at last, the school of nursing came into its own. Adequate scholarship funds were available and a student loan fund had been set up with a Federal Nurses' Training Act grant in 1965. Although there were rumblings on the national scene concerning more education for nurses, hospital diploma schools were still providing most bedside nurses and their educational programs were improving yearly. Ours had an excellent reputation and could select from a steady stream of applicants. The school received a six-year accreditation in 1966, one of only two New Hampshire schools to attain such accreditation from the National League for Nursing, but the faculty was not content with this approval and began considering curriculum revision at the end of the year.

After attending the National League for Nursing meeting with Kathleen Clare at which the nursing hierarchy recommended associate and bachelor's degrees for nurses, Norman Brown reported on a meeting the nursing school committee and an ad hoc committee advising nursing service had held. A discussion of the direction nursing education should take resulted in the consensus that the hospital's school ought to step up its recruiting to make ours the strongest diploma school possible until the direction of change became clearer. The ad hoc committee, looking at ways to improve staffing at the hospital, had explored recruitment possibilities, concluding that their best source of nurses was their own school which would provide twenty-seven new nurses (from a class of twenty-nine) at graduation in 1967, many of whom were interested in those hard-to-fill night and weekend shifts.

These were the best years of the school's history when the school taught large classes of enthusiastic young women. One class during this period, that of 1964, produced three nurses who later returned to teach at the school. Mary Rosa Duprey (McGilvray) returned in 1968 to teach fundamentals of nursing and later maternal-child nursing. She had served as a medical-surgical nurse at the hospital, had done private duty nursing and worked

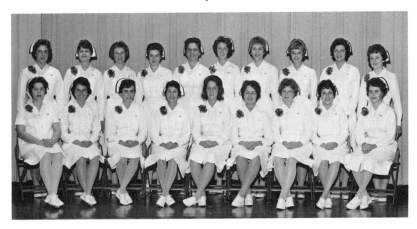

The class of 1964 in a graduation portrait taken in the new school auditorium. Pat Tobin is third from left, Mary Duprey McGilvray and Linda Rule Blais third and second from right in first row.

at a nursing home, along the way earning a B.S. in psychology/sociology. Linda Rule (Blais) was a staff nurse and relief supervisor in the operating room after her graduation. She worked for a group medical practice then returned to the school to teach operating room nursing in 1982. Her B.S. was earned in psychology/sociology, and at the school's close she is nearing attainment of a master's degree in community health education. Patricia Tobin served as a staff nurse at Concord Hospital and several other hospitals after her 1964 graduation. She returned in 1970 to teach medical-surgical nursing after earning her B.S.N. She became the school's director of admissions in 1969 and has earned a master's degree in education and human services. Tobin has also been the instigator of alumni activities for some years, planning alumni banquets around the annual graduation ceremonies. She has served as the conduit through which countless alumni have kept in touch with their school.

Like the class of 1956, the class of 1964 had two homes. They began school on the hospital's fifth floor where noise was a problem. At first the air conditioning system vibrated so loudly that the students were forced to make even more noise just to be heard. An acoustical ceiling improved the situation, and later baffles were placed on the air conditioning tower because the hospital's neighbors had complained too. These students were a fun-loving group and tales are told of midnight forays down to the operating rooms where, on at least one occasion lobsters were steamed in the autoclave.[4] The

move to the new building must have been a relief on the part of those in
authority for it afforded an opportunity for high jinks in a more appropriate setting.

Traditions came to an end in the late sixties. The medical staff ended its
sponsorship of a spring dance, when, like most young people in the turbu-
lent sixties, the students lost interest in formal affairs.

Donation Day died a natural death in 1967. It simply didn't fit in with
the kind of fund raising that was now being carried out, and chances were
that housewives were no longer spending time over their preserve kettles
in order to have rows of jam jars available for contribution.

Now the hospital had a pension plan for employees and the medical staff
was beginning to acquire the rudiments of a library.

The school changed its program to graduate students in June. As more
academic credits were added to its curriculum, the school like many others
found an academic calendar necessary. A physical education program at
Concord's YMCA for which the faculty had high hopes did not work well
and was abandoned in 1968. That year the State Board of Nursing commented in its approval of licensure that the school had the best facilities in the
state, the same opinion held by the federal government's inspector upon completion of the building.

At this juncture hospital trustees were considering plans for the institution's future, one direction being a change in orientation to make the hospital
part of an extended care facility, to be constructed by the Sheraton Corporation. Trustees realized that outside consultation would be advantageous
in formulating plans for the future and hired the firm of Dr. Anthony J.
Rourke to study this issue and others.

Dr. Charles Macomber was appointed to the obstetric-gynecology staff
in 1968, the year that Peter Booth, a graduate of the University of Minneso-
ta's program in hospital administration arrived to aid Administrator Norman Brown and his Assistant Administrator Ella Siegler. This was also the
year that the medical staff asked trustees to ban the sale of cigarettes in the
hospital, a sensitive issue that the board managed to table until 1971, finally voting to ban the sale in the Hospitality Shop when the stock on hand
was depleted. Regulations on smoking were to become far more stringent
in the eighties. At one point the administrator reminded physicians that they
were among the most flagrant violators of these regulations.

During 1970 and 1971 plans were underway for a major expansion of the
hospital by means of a $3 million dollar renovation and construction pro-
gram to increase bed capacity from 195 to 232. Among the areas to be ad-

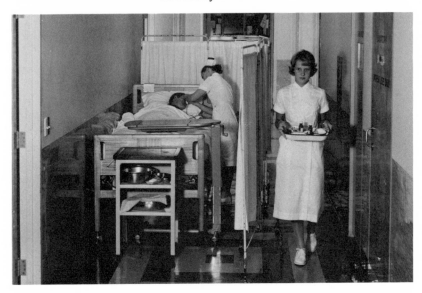

A crowded corridor underscores the need for expansion faced by a fast growing hospital at the end of the sixties when it was little more than ten years old.

dressed in this phase I of a longterm expansion plan were those needed badly by the auxiliary: an office for the volunteer director, a gift shop and additional snack bar space. Administration's needs for office space were acute, as were those of the dietary and pharmacy areas. The medical staff had campaigned for and were eagerly looking forward to an intensive care unit that would also serve coronary patients. The laboratory was in need of space as was the radiology department. Virtually the entire operation would be renovated and reorganized with this expansion.

The staff was enlarging with a new radiologist, R. King Warburton, a new speciality area, that of neurosurgery, to be performed by Merwyn Bagan, and a new controller, Richard Fredrickson. Dr. Philip Boulter arrived in Concord in June, 1971 as a locum tenens and he and his wife Suzanne Boulter, a pediatrician, joined the staff the following year.

The school of nursing had broadened the composition of its advisory committee. Elaine Hoyt, who had joined the school in 1954 was placed on the committee as the school's educational director. A nurse educator from a program other than the Concord Hospital school as well as a representative of a community health agency (replacing a public health nurse) were added. The school's affiliation with Boston's Children's Hospital was dis-

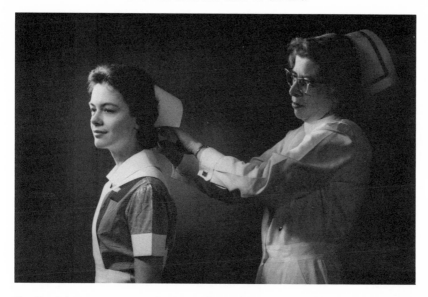

Kay Yeaple became expert over the years in the correct method of pinning on a cap. Here she provides the first symbol of the nursing profession for Helen Marden at the capping ceremony in 1971.

continued and new local affiliations were under scrutiny.

Men were admitted to the school for the first time. Three young men entered the school in 1971, but no men successfully completed the program (most failed academically) until 1976 when William Brothers and Kenneth Forcier were graduated.

For the first time in New Hampshire a bond issue would finance the hospital's expansion. Legislation was passed creating the New Hampshire Higher Educational and Health Facilities Authority which issued the bonds for phase I of the long range expansion.

The hospital adopted its statement on free care in 1972 as a consequence of receiving Hill-Burton funds in 1956 and 1962 for construction. Acceptance of those federal grants required recipients to select from three options. Concord Hospital's trustees selected the option which inspired the following statement: "It is the established policy of Concord Hospital to provide services on the sole basis of the medical necessity for such services as determined by the medical staff without reference to race, color, ethnic origin, creed, sex, or inability to pay for such service." This policy is in effect today.

The trustees lost through retirement, Franklin Hollis and I. Reed Gourley,

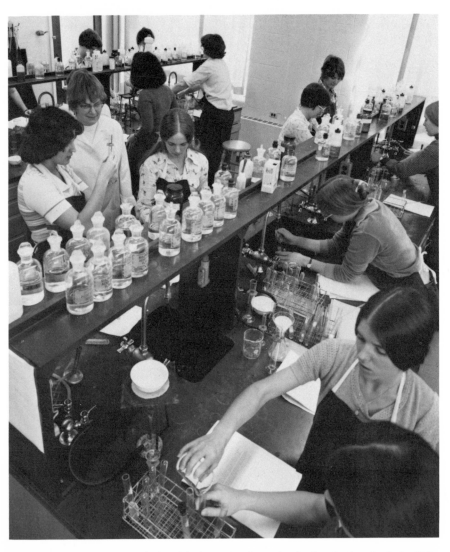

Noel Grossman instructs a microbiology lab class in this photo taken for the school catalog in the 1970s.

two men who had served for many years, and Jane Sanders, a thirteen-year trustee and secretary of the board, who died.

The school, preparing for what became a successful visit from the National League for Nursing, was also engaged in an effort to recruit minority students. Alas, the effort failed, for in the twenty high schools visited that year there were only forty minority students, none of whom were contemplating nursing careers.

In 1972 the school of nursing applied for its first grant from the Helene Fuld Health Trust. The trust (the story of which deserves a history of its own) was established by an eccentric New Yorker, Leonhard Fuld, who with his sister Florentine amassed a respectable fortune from investments in Harlem tenements. He lived in one himself, often serving as janitor. His canny investments enabled him to found a trust in 1969 with assets of over $41 million dollars, its chief beneficiaries to be schools of nursing.[5] Administered by the Marine Midland Bank of New York City, the trust made grants in 1987 of nearly $3 million dollars to 58 schools in addition to funding an NLN accreditation outcomes study, a series of videotapes on nursing theorists, and a grant to the National Student Nurses' Association.

In 1973, the trustees accepted the first grant to our school in the amount of $25,000 for audiovisual equipment. Over the years there have been many other grants from Helene Fuld including monies for the remodelling of the school building adding additional classrooms, air conditioning for the school, a station wagon for students to use when travelling to affiliations, the school's closed circuit security system, radio page units for clinical instructors, and additional audiovisual aids. The school's word processor represents the most recent grant of this unusual trust.

Charles Toll was the new board president in 1973. His first duty was to express the appreciation of his fellow trustees for years of dedicated service to Justice Lawrence I. Duncan, who had been a trustee for 26 years, and to J. Richard Jackman, retiring president, who had guided the institution through its recent enlargement.

The hospital had problems with inflation in 1974 as did the ordinary citizen. Heating oil had risen in cost by 300 percent and dairy products and operating room supplies had skyrocketed. Expense projections were rendered useless. Fortuitously, a rate increase became possible even though the government's economic stabilization program had placed a moratorium on rate increases. Because the hospital had increased the value of its plant by more than 70 percent with its building program, it was entitled to the status of a new facility.

The medical staff that year voted to recommend paid emergency room

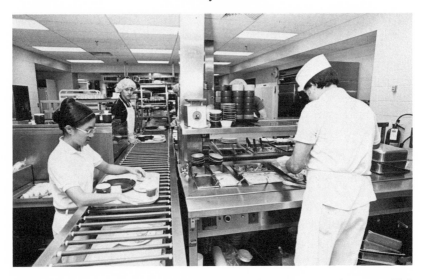

Behind the scenes in the hospital's dietary department. Patients' trays are being assembled before transfer in heated carts to the units.

physicians to replace the on-call rotation system they had employed since the earliest years. Four physicians could provide 24-hour coverage of the emergency room.

The modular building that now rests behind the nursing school as a carpentry and maintenance shop, earlier office space for the school of nursing, was constructed in 1974 to provide space for mental health therapy and patient recreation. Called the Activity Center it was located where the present patient tower is and moved when that phase of expansion began in the early eighties.

In February 1975 Peter Booth left the hospital and Richard Warner arrived in May to assist Norman Brown with his growing work load. He had been administrator at Exeter Hospital and had the reputation as an effective negotiator with third party payers. This kind of expertise was increasingly necessary as each contract with Blue Cross-Blue Shield now took months to negotiate.

The hospital was involved for some time in the acquisition of the tract of land with a house which lay directly adjacent to its property on the east. The property had been part of the Christian Scientists' holdings and had been sold to a group of physicians without notice to the hospital. The group found it difficult to design an office building on the site owing to insurmount-

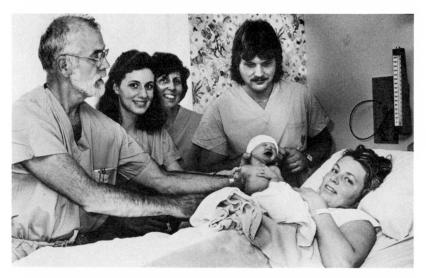

Birth is a family event at Concord Hospital. Dr. Douglas Black presides over a delivery witnessed by the infant's father, grandmother and a Dartmouth medical student.

able traffic problems. Ironically, traffic problems were the reason the hospital needed the land. In the next phase of expansion a new driveway entrance to the hospital would be needed. On the west side of the Pleasant Street property, concern is periodically expressed for the plan, on the city's maps for years, to construct a by-pass highway which would cross the hospital's land. The hospital has been repeatedly assured that this is a low priority with the state highway department, but the question persists. Two other acquisitions long planned for did not come to pass. The hospital was unable to purchase the Christian Science retirement home when the state decided to sell it, and the board spent many fruitless hours as did the hospital's administrative staff in an effort to have the new state neuropsychiatric hospital located on Concord hospital's campus. Today it rises on the former golf course at the old state hospital.

While preliminary plans for expansion were underway, new innovations were engaging the attention of hospital personnel. The lengthy application process to acquire a CAT (computerized axial tomography) scanner was initiated. Dr. Ford von Reyn, a specialist in infection control arrived and emergency room physicians began teaching a group of paramedic students in an emergency medical technician program in conjunction with the New Hampshire Technical Institute. Drs. Walter Dueger and Munro Proctor inaugu-

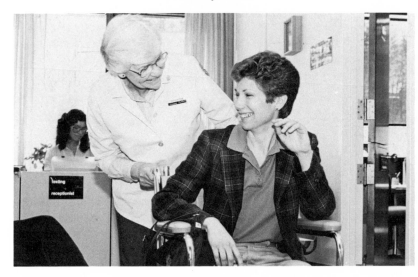

Joanne Teague exemplifies the friendly concern of the hospital volunteer. Her many hours of work were recognized in 1988 when she received the American Hospital Association's volunteer award.

rated the hospital's department of cardiology.

Early in 1977 Norman Brown had announced his intention to retire in July. It was the sense of the trustees that Richard Warner should become the next administrator and they made his appointment official on January 17, 1977. In May Robert E. Knapp arrived to become an assistant administrator.

Norman Brown's retirement party on June 8 at the Highway Hotel was a family affair, for he had been very popular with everyone who worked at the hospital. Among the gifts presented to him was a graduation award in his name to be presented to a student in the school of nursing who most nearly exemplified the qualities of warmth and understanding which he possessed. Brown claimed that he was retiring to do a little lobstering on the coast, but in reality he had already agreed to serve as a consultant for the hospital and he made many trips to Concord during the expansion years.

The school of nursing faculty spent many hours in 1977 defining student rights, establishing a policy for hearings and appeals, and delineating faculty rights and responsibilities and standards of conduct for students. Early in 1978 the school developed an ethical practice policy regarding information to be printed in the school catalog, student handbook, and in policies on admission and recruitment of students.

David Souter, a superior court judge who became a New Hampshire Su-
preme Court justice assumed the board presidency when Charles Toll resigned. Souter had served as secretary of the board for several years. His
meticulous notes are a joy to read.

In light of the expansion of the hospital which this time would be a major construction program and total renovation of the existing plant, the
building committee began interviewing architects in early 1978 to work with
the Turner Construction Company, already selected. The firm of Pacquette
Associates was chosen to design the project, to cost in excess of $16.5 mil-
lion dollars. The hospital would have 295 beds, about 280 of them in a new
patient tower. Ernst and Ernst was engaged in a feasibility study for the budg-
et and finance committee, and in preparation for a capital campaign the
hospital stopped its yearly solicitation of municipalities within its service
area. Ketchum, Inc. would handle the behind-the-scenes work on the drive.
Richard Patterson was hired in 1978 as director of development and, at first,
community relations. He developed the hospital's planned giving program
and worked with fund raisers, retiring in 1987.

Early planning had proven important for the acquisition of the CAT scanner which took almost three years. When the scanner was finally in place
at the end of 1979, it quickly proved to be of great diagnostic value, many
more patients than had been estimated using it within a few months of its
arrival.

Three retirements occurred in 1978 that changed the character of the
hospital forever. Eileen Wolseley, having served as director of nursing service
since the fifties, left in September. Ella Siegler, assistant administrator, had
left in June after a thirty-five year career beginning as secretary to the administrator, ending as assistant administrator. She is today a wearer of the
pink smock as Thursday's cashier in the Hospitality Shop. The hospital's
longest-ranking employee, Esther Holt, a pioneer medical records librarian, had come to work for Margaret Pillsbury Hospital in July 1928. At her
retirement dinner in December 1978 she was made an honorary member of
the medical staff, perhaps an ironic award to one whose most difficult task
was to induce physicians to complete their charts on time.

Much of 1978 was devoted in the nursing school to the preparation of
a self-evaluation report to be used by the accreditation team who visited the
school in January, 1979. A lengthy report, 161 pages, its preparation took
14 faculty meetings. At that time there were 108 students in the school, more
than the number for which the building had been designed. Seventy-nine
students lived in the residence wings, twenty-nine commuted. The faculty's
careful preparation of the report coupled with the results of the visit earned

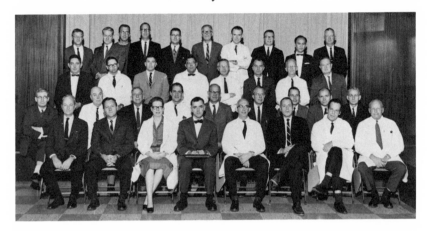

Obstetrician-gynecologist Douglas Black, front row center, was president of the medical staff in 1980 when they sat for this portrait. John Branson, internist, front row right end, died that year.

the school a full eight-year accreditation.

Guests attending a special meeting of the board of trustees in June, 1978 were there to explain the Community Health Study to be conducted with funds from the Jessie Gould Trust through the New Hampshire Charitable Fund. Frank Foster, M.D., an internist with 50 years of medical practice would be working with a five-person citizen's committee to study the delivery of health care in New Hampshire, specifically in the area covered by Concord Hospital. Those conducting the study hoped to use information contained in reports and studies conducted by the hospital and others. The hospital agreed to cooperate extensively with the survey team whose report, issued in 1980 validated the hospital's own expansion plan. The surveyors, however, were somewhat disturbed with the complacency of the Concord community with regard to its own health care, evidenced by lack of interest in the six public forums conducted as part of the survey.[6]

Planning the expansion was now in high gear as a Certificate of Need application was filed with the two agencies regulating hospitals, the Office of Health Planning and Development and the United Health Systems Agency. The administrator began talks with the Concord Steam Corporation which wanted to run a steam line from its State Hospital plant to the hospital entrance where the hospital would take over with a feeder line to the new building. Though the idea appeared to be a good one, no phase of construction proved more troublesome, the entire process becoming a cliffhanger as the building neared completion without a steam line. Eventually the problems, mostly owing to financial difficulties faced by the Steam Corporation, were worked out, and runners who jog along Pleasant Street today can thank the underground line for a clear path even when the snow is deep elsewhere.

Horace Blood, M.D., led the $2 million dollar campaign in 1980. Diligent work with initial givers had assured $1.5 million at the opening dinner held at Bishop Brady High School on March 26, at which not even a bomb scare could dim the attendees' enthusiasm for the task at hand.

One nearby resident who objected to the campaign and building program was Oliver Fifield of Canterbury, who wrote to the hospital as president of Blue Cross-Blue Shield. He asked New Hampshire hospitals to call a moratorium on building projects stating that " . . . it seems obvious that many projects now being planned are part of a competitive race to either preserve a certain level of patient income or to expand at the expense of neighboring institutions. I respectfully suggest that this is a time for hospital trustees to reassess the need to grow bigger at the expense of anyone, especially the consumers of health care."[7]

The expansion program was more than half completed at the time of the dedication of the new patient tower on May 15, 1982. It has been wonderfully described by Justice Souter in his 1981-82 report to the community.

It was a beautiful spring day. Old friends and servants of the hospital came back, neighbors showed up, anyone who could get out of the building for a few minutes did, and it turned into a family party. The Concord High School Brass Ensemble made music before the formalities and Joseph Foley played the national anthem while Mr. Warner raised the flag that Senator Warren Rudman had brought from the capitol in Washington. The president of the Long Island College Hospital in New York, Mr. James Kingsbury, spoke to us; he said the responses to the economic problems of health care had better come from Concord, New Hampshire, and places like it, not from Congress or bureaus in Washington. He didn't have to make any converts. I think, though, he quickened the faith. When the remarks were over we went through the building and had cake and punch out in the afternoon sun.

Justice Souter had begun that annual report with the news that the school of nursing would continue. It had been the subject of a year-long study by the advisory committee of the school under the direction of William A. Oates, rector of St. Paul's School and an overseer of Harvard. Student enrollment was dropping and the hospital's subsidization of the school had grown larger. The committee's report, issued on May 1982 recommended that the school continue to operate as a diploma-granting institution, with

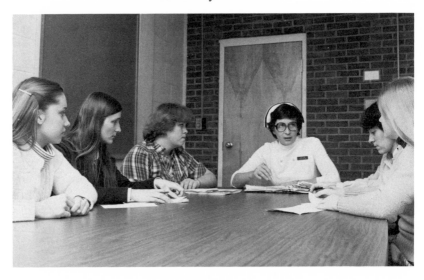

Students discuss the cases they will encounter on patient units in a pre-clinical conference with instructor Caryl Lajoie, a 1959 graduate.

provision for more college credits potentially transferrable to a bachelor's degree. The board of trustees accepted the Oates report and that fall adopted a recommendation from the hospital's development committee to solicit funds on behalf of the school which would strengthen its capital base. The school had already added additional college credits to those offered previously.

Dr. Robert Rainie, retired after 30 years' service on the medical staff, agreed to sign the letter of solicitation, but he did much more than that, taking an active role in the campaign, writing personal notes of thanks for contributions. Beginning slowly, the campaign became quite successful. The school had much to thank Dr. Rainie for, most visibly, scholarship money to keep students in school, audiovisual equipment and a computer for student instruction, and a badly needed photocopier employed by students and faculty alike. He was presented a resolution of thanks at the school's 1986 graduation ceremony held at Memorial Hall, St. Paul's School.

In his last report to the community David Souter paid tribute to Kathleen Clare Yeaple's more than thirty years of able work as director of the school of nursing. She retired in December 1983 and in the witty cogent style so typical of the writing of this brilliant justice he characterizes Yeaple's

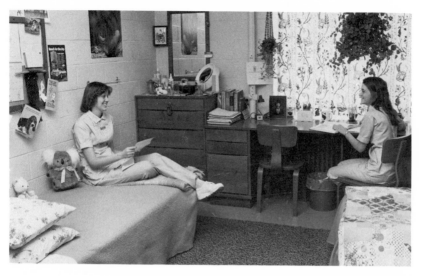

The dormitory wings of the new nursing school building provided cozy accommodations for students who lost no time in creating a "home away from home" atmosphere.

tenure: "Without her, probably ours would have followed the many other hospital schools that closed over the last decade. But she was here and the school she leaves can only live up to her by demanding excellence and getting it, as she has done."

Elaine M. Hoyt followed Kay Yeaple in a seamless transition that could only have occurred between two people who had worked together for many years. As educational director and an instructor in the school since 1954, Hoyt was able to continue the school's demand for excellence in clinical performance and academic work from its students. Indeed, this demand has most likely been a reason for the high attrition rate of beginning students coupled with the program's requirement that students start their work on patient units a brief six weeks after they arrive as freshmen. Students face the reality of nursing quickly, and for some comes the realization that nursing is not to be their career.

Between 1981 and 1984 more than physical growth was taking place at the hospital. The regulatory bodies began to create problems with the acquisition of major equipment, the CAT scanner, then MRI (magnetic resonance imaging) and lithotripsy (the bombardment of kidney stones with sound waves). The dreaded DRGs, or diagnosis related groups arrived to

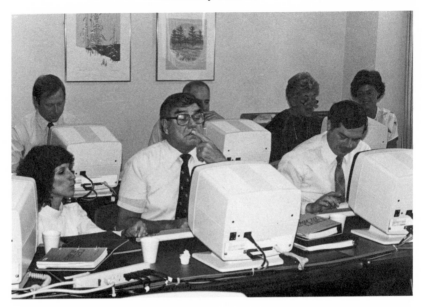

The administrative team is the most recent department to embrace computer technology. Here an instructor observes as Richard Warner ponders the correct command to send a message.

plague the medical staff in 1984. The hospital retained the services of Edgar Helms, former commissioner of health and welfare for the state, to advise on the bewildering array of outside influences which encroach on the daily existence of hospitals.

About two years of study and consultation were required before the hospital was able to hit back, as many hospitals were doing, with a complete reorganization of the institution's corporate structure to create a holding company which would serve as the parent organization for the nonprofit Concord Hospital, Inc. and one or more for-profit corporations which could become creative as well as competitive in offering new services to the community and drawing area. Ropes and Gray of Boston handled the legalities of the matter, as it had for some sixty-five other New England hospitals.

Capital Region Healthcare Corporation was the name chosen for the parent organization. Trustees and department heads attended educational sessions throughout 1984 to be ready for the vote to be taken at the January 21, 1985, annual meeting. Trustees would be repositioned among the new corporations according to their areas of interest and knowledge. The existing hospital corporation was renamed to become the holding corporation

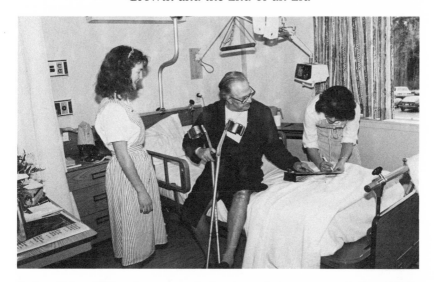

Kathryn Hok and Hillary James were volunteers in a patient care program in the mid-1980s when teens were trained to handle some of the non-nursing tasks necessary in patient care.

and a new hospital corporation was created. The hospital's operating assets (equipment, accounts receivable, etc.) were transferred to the new Concord Hospital corporation. The buildings and land, however, were not transferred because the state would have levied a real estate transfer tax of over $250,000. At present they are leased by the holding company with an option to purchase held by the hospital. A recently purchased parcel of twenty-five acres (the Walker property north of the hospital land) and two smaller buildings (the Burgess house west of the hospital and the day care center, east) along with the hospital's endowment were retained by the holding corporation.[8] Richard Warner was named president and chief operating officer of Concord Hospital, Inc. David H. Rogers became chairman of the board of Capital Region Healthcare Corporation.

Bruce Clow, now president of the hospital board of trustees called the attention of the public to the more than able handling of the intricate processes required in the reorganization by David Rogers during his three-year presidency. Recognition came from his trustee colleagues as well when Rogers was named recipient of the Trustee of the Year award by the New Hampshire Hospital Association.

During and after the reorganization hospital staff members were involved in the development of a number of new services to improve the delivery of

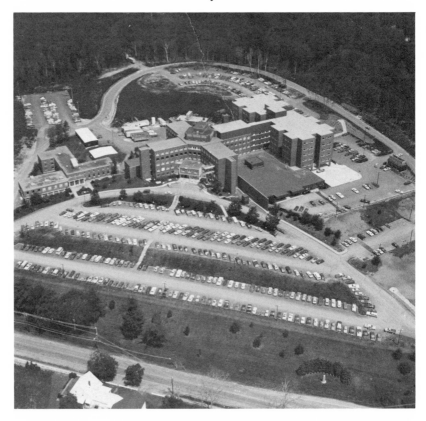

The Concord Hospital campus in the mid 1980s showing the Bradley monument at lower right.
A physicians' office building has recently been erected at top center, and the helipad adjoins
the parking lot, which now fills every available inch of the property.

health care, most prominently a newly designed day surgery center, a walk-in
care center which would free the emergency room for real emergencies and
a second or satellite walk-in care center on Concord Heights. A self-contained
psychiatric unit was opened, the mammography section of the radiology
department modernized and made more responsive to the needs of wom-
en. A second mammography unit opened on the Heights. Joint ventures with
other hospitals were undertaken in the areas of diabetes care, lithotripsy,
and magnetic resonance imaging, the latter two examples of cooperation
bringing the machines in giant eighteen-wheel trailers to the hospitals of the
Merrimack Valley in three-month rotations.

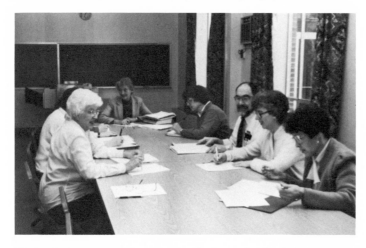

The faculty began meeting every two weeks during the school's last year. Here the group reviews the policy on record retention at a Monday afternoon session.

One example of the benefits of reorganization is the affiliation of the Concord Regional Visiting Nurse Association under the umbrella of the hospital's parent organization. This affiliation, accomplished after study by both boards, will make possible greater efficiency in the coordination and delivery of home care services and makes formal an alliance that has existed for some years with the provision of discharge services purchased from the VNA by the hospital as far back as the sixties.

And finally, the hospital's day care center has been open for two years, a valued benefit for employees and a powerful recruitment lure to potential employees.

The climate has changed from the day in 1984 when the hospital was able to lower daily room rates by $15 to the present struggle for income with patient reimbursement by third party payers deteriorating. A new physicians' office building rises behind the hospital in an effort to produce a new source of income, while down the hill a producer of nurses for the past hundred years prepares to close.

The nursing school committee was requested to make a determination on the future of the school early in 1985 by the board of trustees. Under the direction of former state planner and state senator Mary Louise Hancock, the committee began its deliberations with the 1982 Oates report. As the year progressed it became evident that the class entering in September, 1986

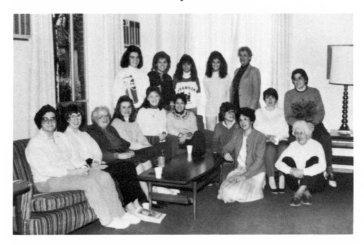

The faculty and members of 1989's class gathered monthly for coffee and conversation in the school living room, an enjoyable break not possible when the school had more than one hundred students.

would be a very small one. Richard Warner wanted the board of trustees to make the decision at its fall meeting in order that recruitment of students could either begin or cease.

Regretfully, the recommendation of the nursing school committee was that the school be phased out, to close upon graduation of the class of 1989. This decision was approved by the board of trustees on October 20, 1986.

As these final words are being written, the faculty and administration have accomplished much of the work involved in closure. They elected to prepare for and host the National League for Nursing's accreditation visit in early 1987 which granted the school full accreditation for the balance of its existence. A closing report was prepared for the League in March 1988, and courses and faculty assignments have been arranged for the final class. A committee on record retention has spent two years devising a policy for the retention of student and school records with procedures for obtaining transcripts as well as caps and replacement pins. Help with emotional reactions to the close was provided faculty and students by hospital counsellors, but the best advice came from Hilda Batchelder, a retired nursing educator who had participated in two school closings. She visited the school for a warmly received question and answer session in early 1987.

The students handled the news well, most expressing their thankfulness that they had arrived at the school just in time, for they were certain that the program suited their needs. Such were the thoughts of Marjorie DuBois, a member of the class of 1988, who had raised ten children before she was able to gratify her lifelong wish for a nursing education, which for her, did not include a degree.[9]

Faculty members were reassigned and most have found other positions in the hospital, a few have changed careers and others are making career decisions now.

Ahead is the last graduation, a happy time for students for whom it is truly a commencement, a sad time for faculty who have been with the school for many years, and a milestone in the history of Concord Hospital.

Epilogue

_____

A story is not worth the telling unless we understand its lesson. This particular lesson is that there is value in remembering the past. Our school of nursing is not just a quaint relic of earlier times, but part of the history of health care without which the modern hospital could not have been born.

Concord Hospital's school and its antecedents represent the best education possible for nurses, each in its own time providing staff nurses for the hospital and others across the country and abroad, school nurses, community health nurses, nurse educators, nursing managers and entrepreneurs, missionary nurses, industrial nurses, military nurses in four wars, and a great many nurses who have raised healthier families as a result of their training.

We are uncertain of the future of nursing, that is, of its future direction, but we do know that people will continue to need care-givers who have been trained to administer whatever form of care is prevalent at the time, employing whatever technology man has devised. We are proud of our history and to have been part of the evolutionary process of health care in Concord, New Hampshire from November, 1889 to May 1989.

> All things change and we must change with them.
>
> --Lothair, ca. 840 A.D.

APPENDICES

Graduates of the Margaret Pillsbury General Hospital School of Nursing

1890
Mary E. Chadwick
Margaret H. Mitchell
Mary Stillings

1891
Margaret Laird

1892
Mary Danforth
Lulu M. Colcord
Edith Foss
Jennie Moulton

1893
Florence E. Anderson
N. Velona Curtice

1894
Lura Jackman
B. Montross Truesdell
Adruenna Allen Tupper
May Wayman

1895
Susan S. Mooney

1896
Laura S. Lohnes
Agnes Robb
Emma J. Rushby

1898
Marion B. Robinson
Eva Sanborn
Dora Whitcher

1899
Louise I. Chase
Ray Cole Heywood
Isabel Nicholson
Ella N. Sanborn

1900
Edna M. Lucas

1901
Catherine Carroll
Etta Beane Huzzey

1902
Bertha M. Clark

Mary Alice Gates
Glenna May G. Morrill
Mabel St. Denis

1903
Catherine R. Cooper
Mary E. McDonald
Elizabeth M. Murphy
Marie Beauclerk Templeton

1904
Bessie H. Clay
Lucy I. Daly
Lucy C. Phillips

1905
Eva St. C. Harris
Marie C. Hodgdon
Margaret R. McCormack
Maud G. Mooney
Della E. Streeter

1906
Ida B. Graham
Margaret M.W. Hartwell
Florence B. Hill
Helena Hogan
Eldya McLean
Gertrude M. Walker

1907
Bertha Craig
Cassie M. Hall
Marion Sullivan Ladd
Eleanor Martin
Grace G. Mundell
Etta Peever
Melanie Rogier

1908
Celia Frances Davis
Katherine A. Grace
Wilhelmina R. Ley
Ethel Peppard
Vinnie M. Randall

1909
Amy Estella Cotton
Marion Jane Kirby
Bessie Millar

1910
Viola Caldwell
Madeline Major
Ethel Emma Richardson
Jennie Ross
Bertha M. Samson
Jane W. Weston

1911
Estelle Maude Bennett
Minnie Hurn
Thurza Brown Jackson
Louisa Pearse
Katherine M. Piper
Ella Blanche Stafford
Nina Winch

1912
Ruth Blanche Allen
Madeline L. Currier
Mae Daniels

1913
Mary Melanson
Jennie M. Peterson
Margaret Robins
Anna L. Scott
Bessie L. Sherlock

1914
Josephine Barrett
Nina Batchelder
Hilma Jeanson
Agnes Ursula Joyce
Mabel Magee

1915
Eleanor Burdette Clough
Beryl DuBoyce
Mildred Tabor

1916
Edith Burgess
Phoebe U. Crosby
Ethel M. Dagles
Ida M. Dawson
Ina M. Deming
Emma Dyson
Myrtle MacAloney
Beatrice Pearce
Viola Stanley

1917

Minnie Avonson
Arlene R. Barrett
Rose Brown
Mabel T. Morse
Nellie Perkins

1918

Bernice E. Driver
Nina M. Hodgdon
Lydia Rivest
Josephine Searles
Mary Grace Wells
Frances Young

1919

Marion Bergeron
Nina B. Clark
Constance B. Eldridge
Florence A. Flanders
Winifred Grant
Alicia Mae Keller
Maude Tilton
Mamie Whyte

1920

Sylvia F. Deane
Hazel O. Ferns
Ruth L. Hinton
Mary L. Huckins
Alice E. Russ
Mable V. Smith

1921

Ruth B. Canfield
Mary A. Hyland
Margaret Eva Lawler
Anna LeBlanc
Leona Rainey
Martha Ross

1922

Ruth L. Gilman
Mary E. Haselton
Mae E. Jewett
Elsie Yetman

1923

Una S. Fuller
Florence Hardy
Grace W. Stevens
Jessie Stewart
Lillian W. Williamson

1924

Priscilla Adams
Addie Gavel
Marian M. Hirtle
Elsie M. Jones
Blanche McFadden

1925

Beatrice Lyford
Alta MacDonald
Frances Irene MacDonnell
Agnes Theriault

1926

Ethel M. Grant
Muriel Philbrick
Janie Rankin Oliver
Abbie S. Tucker

1927

Margaret Faucher
Ida Almira Lovering
Mary Merrick
Lillian Rankin
Mary A. Quimby
Vera Warren

1928

Lillian A. Anderson
Caroline Oldham
Wilda Torrance

1929

Ruth G. Inman
Ethel V.M. Johnson
Gertrude Roselle

1930

Florence E. Berry
Alice Katherine Dudley
Helen F. Dudley
Lucille DuPont
Beatrice MacLean
Mildred Mallory
Frances Martin
Margaret Pickard
Madaline Pierce
Grace G. Rollins
Helen E. Tasker

1931

Evelyn Lois Brown
Doris Flora Ellinwood
Margaret Leonard

Aline Angelina Luneau
Inez Stevenson
Erma Stewart
Mildred Katherine Veino

1932

Edith Frances Chamberlain
Elva Lena Erhart
Emily Harriet Foss
Lillian Maude Hickey
Velma Louise Hutt
Ruth Amanda Morin
Genevieve Monica Mullen
Gladys Abbie Nelson
Frances Philbrick
Mabel Elizabeth Read
Bernice Annie Robertson

1933

Harriet Louise Clark
Edith Fronia Fowler
Olive Jacobs Mitchell
Donna Elizabeth Morrison
Edna Bessie Nelson

1934

Katharine Anne Burke
Arleen Natalie Merrill
Elna Carolyn Messer
Katherine Edith Wood

1935

Florence O. Benoit
Miriam Irene Brunel
Frances Amanda Carleton
Ruth Helen Hagar
Catherine Vanlora Kimball
Emma Levesque
Nancy Abi Young

1936

Phyllis Edith Bushey
Harriet Gertrude Coxon
Alice Gertrude Crane
Beryl Sherman Cummings
Shirley Eunice Tillotson
Harriet Alice Wilkinson

1937

Louise Bartlett
Mamie Rachael Bucklin
Lavona Mura Fifield
Arline Morrison Park
Mary Lela Parkhurst

Charlotte Rebecca Robinson
Ruth Evelyn Westcott
Ernesta Helen Wooster

1938

Priscilla Bragdon
Gertrude Harriet Caldwell
Mabel Roberta Cressy
Ruth Emma Floyd
Phyllis Effie George
Jean Hood
Ula Claire Libby
Elizabeth Minahan
Warancia Motowylak
Ruth Pratt
Arlyne Mildred Roache
Helen Constance Sargeant
Helen Lucy Shlaitas
Irvena Stevens
Marjorie Leona Taylor
Lucy Ann Tsarides
Della Faith Wilson

1939

Helen Grace Atwood
Ruth Lela Bickford
Dorothy Mae Chandler
Sylvia Coy
Margaret Grace Deighton
Vurlyne A. Ellsworth
Carrie B. Gilman
Louise A. Lucas
Audrey Pearl Maguire
Lucy Eleanor Manix
Eunice Newhall
Ruth Ricard
Emily Clara Wood

1940

Marguerite Frances Fogg
Catherine Alice Guertin
Doris Emma Heath
Ethel Cecilia Kimball
Mae Louise Mansfield

Elva Preble Noyes
Amelia Mary Pietraallo
Margaret Anna Sherry
Evelyn Marston Smith
Helen Grace Travis
Rosamund Myra Warren
Florence Ella Webster

1941

Lillian Gertrude Brainerd
Marion Gertrude Crockett
Bertha Agnes Currier
Ruth Eleanor Hamilton
Ruth Emma Hatch
Evelyn May Hugron
Georgia Thelma Mills
Mary Frances Moorenovich
Doris Eva Perkins
Cynthia Perry
Margaret Maria Putney
Flora Alice Young

1942

Cynthia Naomi Crosby
Rachel Madlyn Duprey
Edith Frances Floyd
Carolyn Julianna Lacross
Agnes Frances Rogers
Mary Elizabeth Tibbetts
Virginia Mary Warren
Ruth Dora Welcom
Cynthia Louise Wiggins
Adella Josephine Wilt

1943

Eveleana Margaret Blake
Helen Daroska
Clarice Harriet Fryer
Frances Horne
Margaret McNally
Marguerite Murray
Sylvia C. Skidmore
Loraine Whitcomb Smith
Eleanor Sweatt

Lois Tash
Shirley Trask

1944

Joan Atwood
Bula Mabel Bailey
Jean P. Beard
Lois G. Carter
Marion Dovhaluk
Beatrice May Gile
Pauline E. Gray
M. Harriet Hills
Virginia Holbrook
Doris E. McGrath
Rosa Marceau
Cora Sweatt

1945

Edna Bertha Crane
Marion Ruth Hayden
Gertrude Mae MacDonald
Margaret McLean Mitchell
Geraldine Mary Reidy
Ruby Elaine Trumbull
Priscilla Eva Turner
Marjorie Gertrude Whitcher

1946

H. Joan Cunningham
Alma Vivian Fluke
Margaret Frances Lacey
Dorothy Marguerite Lear
Doris Veronica McCafferty
Phyllis Eleanor McGregor

1947

Clara Louise Berry
Elizabeth Anne Boynton
Corinne Plummer Gilman
Vera Lucy Hill
Madge Lyon Holbrook
Kathryn May Patterson
Mary Ellen Rogers

Graduates of the
New Hampshire Memorial Hospital School of Nursing

1899
Nora M. Brown

1900
Almah Barter
Eva Crosby
Hattie Liscomb

1901
Mary L. Nichols

1902
Mary L. Baker
Mary E. Kile

1903
Annie W. Brown
Mary Kemp
Grace Lucas
Mary Minnigan

1904
Vera Hewitt
Rose Smith

1905
V. Florence Dunbar
Rosanna O'Donaghue
Mary Smith

1906
Blanche Caldwell Atwood
Anna F. McDerby

1907
Ella F. Burke
Etta Doherty
Ada Howe

1908
Mary Gray Barnard
Mary Gay
Margaret McConnell
Elizabeth McPhee
Addie Moore

1909
Florence Asprey
Iva N. Downs
Annie Pickering

1910
Agnes E. Doherty
Janette Pettigrew
Jean F. Wilson

1911
Minnie Armstrong
Grace M. Colby
Clarice Elliott
Nettie Ewing
Helen M. Flanders
Helen Young Upham

1913
Beulah Bugbee
Florence Bugbee
Grace Gifford
Helen Melanson
Elizabeth Noone

1915
Henrietta Altman
Regina Gavin
Nettie E. Gorham
Beryl Hannant
Leonora Mignault

1916
Louise Moulton Hartshorn
Jennie McVety
Margaret Murphy

1917
Jane Isobel Burtt
Beatrice Elizabeth Forster
E. Pearl Graham
Winifred McVety

1918
Mary Flora Hill
Bertha Nicholson
Blanche Parsons
Edith Ross
Sarah Mary Willette

1919
Sara Melanson

1920
Marjorie L. Carrigan

Evelyn Howe
Wilhelmina Schayltz

1921
Margaret Mary Gilmartin
Ruth M. Hall
Gladys Marcotte
Bertha O'Connell
Anne Shepard
Ruth Wilson

1922
Charlotte Batchelder
Ora Hurd
Emma Melanson
Margaret O'Donnell
Lucy Salt
Margaret Willard

1923
Leah Bradbury
Annie DeBoer
Gladys Melanson
Agnes O'Donnell
Lillian Wright

1924
Donna Lucille Burchard
Ruth Esther Dearborn
Stella LaBrossiere

1925
Beatrice Mae Brown
Ina Marden
Ruby Powers

1926
Josephine Elizabeth Gray
Jean MacMillan
Catherine O'Brien
Dorothy York

1927
Frances Annette Bailey
Ruth Helen Colby
Doris Edith Davis
Linda Belle Farnum
Minnie Evangeline Fulton
Gladys Louise Greeley
Helen Luce
Helen Merriam

Hilda C. Roberts
Lean Uehlein
Dorothea Wheeler

1928

Louise Dekkers
Laura Emma Hayward
Annie Lund
Dorothea O'Neill
Lucy Shepard
Florence Simpson
Edith Wood

1929

Anna Sweeney
Edith Tucker

1930

Jennie Mae Clay
Veronica Rebecca Dion
Carmen Alice Gilbert
Dorothea Margaret
    Goodwin
Lillian May Gordon
Martha Knight
Blanche Reid
Beulah Ethel Wark
Mae Ida Watts
Emma Werner

1931

Olive Beauparlant
Harriet Elizabeth Bryant
Louise Cogger
Irene Gray
Helen Lee
Sylvia McIntosh
Irene O'Donnell
Luella Palmer

1932

Gladys H. Caldon
Edith B. Ebert
Grace Hernandez
Hazel McLaughlin
Myrtle Miller
Eleanor Taylor

1933

Margaret Elizabeth Call
Helen Frances Giblin
Ruth Eleanor Kenney
Kathleen Lane
Helen Stewart

1934

Elizabeth A. Carter
Anna Jean Dever
Dorothy Geneva Fifield
Muriel Whynott

1935

Esther Louise Black
Ethel Chambers
Lorna Coburn
Blanche Foss
Hazel Ethel Haggett
Ruth Knuckey
Mary P. Malone
Lois Saturley
Esther Wright

1936

Mabel L. Carter
Doris Anna Heller
Thelma Frances Hoffman
Frieda Joseph
Adelma Lajoie
Edith Prescott
Mary Ugolnik
Martha Weston

1937

Dorothy Coolong
Gertrude Mae Crosby
Edyth Louise Elliott
Blanche Lucille Falanga
Hazel F. Howard
Mary Theresa Lafley
Pauline B. Simon
Katherine Splane

1938

Thelma Gertrude Baston
Virginia J. Chaplick
Charlotte Theresa Dorin
Cecilia Marguerite Drapeau
Dorothy Mae Hayford
Ruth Jones
Mary Agnes Kuczynska
Dorothy A. Malone
Mabel Peterson

1939

Margaret Levesque
Madeline McMann
Arlene Moore
Alice Ziskind

1940

Barbara Lucille Connary
June Craig
Lydia C. Harris
Violet Keniston
Barbara Nelson

1941

Clara Anna Freeman
Anita Clarice Gold
Marion MacLean
Charlotte L. Mossey
Mildred L. Rush
Barbara Saunders
Stella Sawyer
Esther V. Shackford
Katherine M. Thompson
Natalie Wells
Otelia M. Weschrob

1942

Elizabeth Jane Bagley
Mary Proud Bailey
Mary Celine Blanchard
Edith V. Drake
Virginia B. Keniston
Beatrice Lees
Evelyn Preve
Margaret M. Reardon
Augusta Tuckos

1943

Margaret F. Beals
Margaret Alice Peabody
Eleanor M. Tyrer
Dorothy E. Woodes

1944

Dorothy Pearl Andrews
Katherine Louise Bagley
Jean Crombie
Barbara Robertson
Evelyn Schuman
Shirley Phillips Silver

1945

Edith Rowan Bowden
Carolyn Louise Colby
Claire J. Eggleston
Barbara J. Evans
Catherine Q. Fredette
Arline C. Gifford
Marion L. Hebert

Barbara A. Johnson
Elizabeth Anne Kelley
Blanche E. Knowles
Pearl Melissa Kimball
Rita J. Landry
Edith Paquin
Ruth Evelyn Sanborn
Dorothy Sargent
Norma Augusta
    Schliessman
Helen J. Seabury

1946

Ella Mary Fifield
Marjorie Pauline Fontaine
Irene Griffin
Nancy Healy
Charlotte Lura Matava
Muriel Mary May
Veronica Rita McCarthy
Mary Reese
Leone Richards
Doris Treamer

Barbara Jamesina Wells
Clara Louise Yeaton

1947

Dorothy Barnum
Shirley Louise Bonneau
Pauline L. Clairmont
Barbara J. Goudie
Phyllis S. Hamilton
Ella Severance
Shirley F. Taylor
Marguerite Varotsis

Graduates of the Concord Hospital School of Nursing

SEPTEMBER, 1947

Lois Marilyn Ames
Elizabeth Carol Avery
Dorothy Louise Barnum
Katherine Shirley Boyce
Arlene Louise Butman
Beverly Alice Fisher
Pauline Greene
Bessie Louise Labor
Arlene M. Marston
Dorothy Agnes Marston
Gladys Elaine Owen
Elsie Elaine Pettigrew
Marie Edythe Phillips
Helen Maud Scott
Helen M. Stevens

FEBRUARY, 1948

Ardell Frances Call
Doris Louise Crosscup
Harriet Waterman Currier
Claire Merilyn Dunbar
Edna Jean Kinne
Helen Martha Lambert
Evelyn Laraway
Mary Louise McAuley
Adele Leonarda Ponzio
Mary G. Swinnerton
Elizabeth Tomkinson
Virginia White
Margaret Wunderlich

SEPTEMBER, 1948

Helen Louise Burnham
Janet Ruth DeLysle
Marion Emeline Dorman
Ruthyvonne Fuller
Marilyn Louise Knapton
Bertha Ruth Morse
Joyce Powell
Myrtle Roberts
Lois Ida Willson

FEBRUARY, 1949

Edith Helen Carr
Louise Marie Champagne
Lucille Ryan Kidder
Ethel L. Murray
Gertrude Richards
Florence Springett
Eleanor Turner
Margaret Washburn

Mary E. Whitcomb

SEPTEMBER, 1949

Alice Keeler Clark
Madeline Grace Finley
Ruth Natalie Huntoon
Helen Koutrelakos

FEBRUARY, 1950

Marcelline Eunice Dolloph
Eileen Margaret Dunmore
Irene Helen Sowa

SEPTEMBER, 1950

Nancy Hoit Donnelly
Gloria Elaine Moore
Joan Sawyer

FEBRUARY, 1951

Barbara Louise McLeod
Bernice Joycelyn Macomb
Barbara Ann Marsland

SEPTEMBER, 1951

Lorraine Muriel Beane
Patricia Jane Eastman
Elberta Ruth Farrar
Norma Ann Garvey
Marilyn Priscilla Gates
Virginia Faye Johnson
Kathleen Ann Lachenal
Bernice Emily Moulton
Joan Patricia Rice
Mary Beatrice Stevens
Betty Jane Stratton

FEBRUARY, 1952

Jean Clara Draper
Jean Marion MacKenzie
Ruth Louise Ringland

SEPTEMBER, 1952

Irene Pauline Archambault
Joanne Adelia Austin
Mary Elizabeth Ballard
Beverly Ann Bartkus
Corrine Boudreau
  Cassavaugh
Mary Louise Colby
Alice Eldean Dow
Helen Agnes Flanagan
Barbara Ann Kingsbury
Pauline B. Lugg
M. Thelma Markey

Shirley May Milner
Elsa Emma Renker
Jane Louise Rowe
Avis MacKenzie Skivington
Naida Ann Wells

FEBRUARY, 1953

Jean Smith Aslanian
Gladys Lorraine Briggs
Laura Jean Richdale
Elaine Barbara Seamans
Carole Stenzel Talbott

SEPTEMBER, 1953

Ann Marie Banks
Betty Lou Bennett
Emma Mae Buker
Marilyn Calef
Jacqueline Louise Clay
Barbara Amee Coit
Shirley Warner Dickson
Helen A. Filides
Elizabeth Ann Fiske
Arlene Bertha Gove
Barbara Ann Hilton
Ruth I. Long
Coral Jean Mitchell
Joan Dow Morrill
Marjorie Kathryn Pettes
Jean Marilyn Smith

1954

Mary Ann Axon
Glennis Stewart Baldwin
Priscilla Holmes Basson
Marcia Reinhard Brooks
Florence E. Butler
Marilyn Ina Clement
Janet Griffin Durling
Charlene Mary Flanagan
Elizabeth Mae LaCross
Nanet Evelyn Laflam
Ida Laurina LaMadeleine
Margaret Malitsos
Shirley Lorraine McKenzie
Janice Marie Preve
Effie Jane Watson
Katherine Lydia Wood

1955

Dorothy Thompson Belko
Claudine Hope DeCato
Sylvia West Falzone

Helen Frances Gerrish
Patricia Mae Gray
Phyllis Whynott Morneault
Shirley Westerberg Scribner
Earlah Hayes Swift
Janet Marie Vachon
Agnes Audrey Walwork

1956

Marjorie Esther Ames
Beverly Mae Cleary
Dorothy Ellen Colpitts
Margaret Elizabeth
    Davignon
Alice Ruffle Dutton
Alida Drewry Ferguson
Maxine Lorraine Holt
Judith Ann Marden
Christine Anastasia Niarchos
Ruth Evelyn Perkins
Evelyn Mae Smead
Beverly Ann Stathers
Jane Betty Stevens
Patricia Ann Tilton
Ann Theresa Vincent
Barbara Jane Winkley

1957

Marian Joyce Annis
Anne Bailey
Sandra Bennett Carswell
Mildred Veronica Chacos
Marie Angel Croft
Nancy Lea Follansbee
Jean Irene Gallagher
Judith Foster Garran
Ann Marguerite Gilman
Ann Marie Hilson
Alvienar Ann King
Kathleen Phyllis Martin
Raelene Wood McLain
Marcia Elaine Miles
Arlene Joan Thibeault
Shirley Phyllis Treffrey
Nancy Lea Tuttle
Theresa Yvonne Valorose
Nancy Rice Vigue
Rosemary Nutter Willey
Lorraine Smith Young

1958

Leona Nutter Arata
Ann Heather Burchell

Joan Marie Butler
Janet Laura Carter
Irene Colby Clark
Betsy Renette Earle
Cynthia Richardson Falcetti
Sondra Joan Hussey
Betty Rideout Leaf
Jane Dewey Langill
Barbara Ann Martel
Beverly Gray Miller
Elizabeth Agnes Owen
Emily Ann Owen
Anna Marie Peterson
Gail Lucille Poland
Marilyn Ann Ramsdell
Pauline Eleanor Sherman
Laura Jones Towns
Germaine Baer Whiting
Margaret Jane Woodbury

1959

Kathleen Priscillann Barton
Joyce Marion Batchelder
Sandra Lee Brett
Caryl Louise Burbank
Nancy Ellen Cameron
Laurel Brown Colby
Marlene Shaw Cuthbertson
Kathleen Whitney Daniels
Sonja Elizabeth Davidson
Charlotte Evelyn Davies
Una Joyce Drewry
Mona Lee Gendreau
Rebecca Jean Guyette
Sarah Naomi Hart
Mary Ann Howe
Ann Schofield Huckins
Audrey King Kiepper
Shirley Jean Laughy
Clara Patricia Littlefield
Katherine M. MacIver
Joyce Laware Neveux
Patricia Marie Regent
Barbara May Reid
Mildred Lois Robinson
Marjorie Louise Small
Roberta Ann Southwick
Nancy Trevelyan Whitehill

1960

Edna Marie Adams
Doris Esther Beck
Elise Marie Bernier

Raylene Leona Bradbury
Susan Carolyn Darby
Sandra Lee Dodds
Gail Elaine Forest
Judith Marie Gay
Natalie June Hartwell
Nancy Ann Hohman
Sandra Palmer Howe
Edith Helen Keyser
Kathleen Rose Murphy
Muriel Frances Treffrey
Judith Ann Wells

1961

Rosalie Ann Avery
Theresa Julia-Anne Badger
Evelyn Joann Bordner
Elizabeth Emily Bradbury
Kathryn Edna Moore Combs
Phyllis Theresa Farmer
Judith Fisk Gilmore
Barbara Helen Kelsea
Anne Bradford Leavitt
Ruth Marie Lloyd
Helen Rosalie Marden
Brenda Lois Moore
Maureen Teresa Perry
Judith Ann Questrom
Alinda Gail Roy
Judith Arlene Senter
Harlean Ann Shaw
Joyce Lue Smith
Evelyn Lois Treloar
Diana Jane White
Ethel Grace Woodward
Virginia Estelle Young

1962

Mary Bristol
Yvonne Claveau
Margaret Dunsmore Coon
Ann Elizabeth Daley
Lorraine Velma Gould
Lorna Beatrice Hoitt
Florence Barss Huntington
Elizabeth Ann Huntoon
Judy Lee Jenness
Sandra Jean Lamere
Charlotte Edith Landry
Roberta Elaine Leigh
Louise Betty Malmgren
Anne Marie McGreevy
Marie Paula Najuck

Appendices

Nancy Louise Perkins
Marjorie Ann Smith
Pamela Faye Smith
Carol Ann Thiem
Sally Patch Whitcher
Nancy Delores Willis

1963

Virginia Bartlett Bailey
Susan Jean Beattie
Jacqueline S. Bellefeuille
Rose Mary Guerriero
  Blaisdell
Pamela Gould Chickering
Susan Payne Dalton
Judith Lee Edmunds
Tracy Johnson
Nancy Ruth Kenney
Judith Faulkingham Komarek
Lois Perkins Loomis
Martha Marion Lynch
Dianne MacDougall
Susan Stewart Macey
Dianne Dorene Maratea
Carol Frances McGrath
Joan Amelia McPhail
Carol Crawford Mudgett
Nancy Guimond Mullavey
Lynda Ann Newcombe
Ella May Portigue
Sarah Ann Seavey
Jo-Ann Usko Tinker
Mavourneen Madeline
  Tisdale
Marcia Heard Wadsworth

1964

Karlyne Sudsbury
  Ainsworth
Ann Batchelder
Patricia Johnson Bigwood
Gail Brett
Nancy Reynolds Crepeau
Paula Ann Comtois
Mary Rosa Duprey
Lucinda Greene Gibson
Carolyn Louise Grant
Patricia Ann Hubbard
Jane Kathrine McArdle
Judith Mary Nay
Kathryn Eleanor Papineau
Constance Ellen Richards
Linda Mae Rule

Sandra Shipman
Elinor May Sinclair
Patricia Anne Tobin
Brenda Law Wheeler

1965

Lois Elizabeth Allen
Judith Ann Allison
Cheryl Louise Avery
Ann Collins Cargill
Ellen Anne Clark
Jerritt Bethlyn Dane
Prudence Dale Davis
Joanne Lynne Dietrich
Louise Clara Dupont
Jean Anne Keefe
Jeanne Eleanor Levesque
Karen Muriel Lutze
Linda Lee Marden
Marcia Leah McCann
Donna Lee Merrill
Marjorie Ellen Peck
Katherine Ruth Philbrick
Linda Ann Stancliff
Ann Barbara Taylor
Mary Louise Tibbetts
Ann Theresa Wagner

1966

Marilyn Hurd Barselle
June Carol Benner
Connie Ruth Bogle
Helen Martha Dexter
Linda Olson Gallagher
Irene Judith Garofalo
Vivian Marie Gosselin
Judith Susan Hunt
Eileen Jean Kaczmarski
Judith Ann Kennison
Sharon Ann Lawrence
Susan Alice Lewis
Annette Dodier Lord
Patricia Mary Lowden
Lucille Anita Marquis
Doreeta Florence Meroff
Linda Claire Miller
Jeanne Marie Morin
Victoria Lambert Northcott
Brenda Lee Northup
Kathryn Muriel Ober
Barbara Jean Preston
Barbara Louise Thibault
Ardyce Jane Washburn

Susan Agnes Whitcomb
Cheryle Ann Wood
Alida Campbell Yonchak

1967

Linda Ruth Austin
Jean Ann Bridge
Judith Pearle Brooks
Clare Louise Brown
Janet Evelyn Farnum
Janet Marie Goodhue
Rebecca Ann Hull
Joan Laura Ladieu
Sheryl Ann Lester
Mary Jane Lord
Nancy Lee Madden
Noel Kathryn Mannion
Joni Carole McLaughlin
Theresa Rachael Melville
Elizabeth Jean Nelson
Linda Ann Neuman
Lizabeth Anne Noyes
Susan Betty Ober
Marsha Kay Patterson
Patricia Joann Proulx
Dorothy Miriam Rand
Diana Lynne Runser
Cynthia Ann Tardiff
Nancy Elizabeth Taylor
Marion Louise Valentine
Sharon Kay Van Tassel
Judith Ann Virgin
Sue Carole Weidhaas
Agnes Lillian Wheeler

1968

Dorothy Elaine Aldrich
Jennifer Lee Appleby
Beverly Jean Aubert
Patricia Fiske Baker
Gail Davis Barnes
Margaret Ann Briscoe
Susan Brooke
Jeanne Estella Buzzell
Juanita Chase Caisse
Cassandra Ellen Campbell
E. Mary Carroll
Nancy Louise Davis
Ellen Rose Dutton
Susan Jean Fay
Marilyn Dougherty
  Flannagan
Hazel Mae Forbes

Shirley Walters Freeman
Judith Irene LeMay
Suzanne Patricia Marcou
Diane Claire Muzzey
Kathleen Margaret Spence
Norrine Lee Tefft
Susan Marie Therrien

1969

Susan Hankins Andrews
Linda Jean Beach
Marjorie Alice Black
Judith Anne Blouin
Kathleen Jean Brooks
Joan Dallas Buchan
Frankie May Craig
Norma Rita Cross
Phyllis Louise Donahue
Pamela Elizabeth Fellows
Linda Ann Harbour
Katherine Agnes Kimball
Elaine May LaPan
Marylee Ledger
Elieen Dawn McMullen
Florence Rowell Merrill
Arleen Barbara Mixer
Cathy Lee Perkins
June Smith Puglisi
Lorna Jean Smith
Donna Stevens
Beverly Ann Tessier
Marion Bourque Watrous
Susan Gale Wheeler
Judith Ann Whitcher
Kathryn McCormack Young

1970

Susan Fenno Abbott
Carol Hansen Aspinall
Jennifer Louise Avery
Martha Ann Brown
Catherine Lynn Carlisle
Julia Ann Chaykowsky
Beverly Ann Coutts
Barbara Jean Cowling
Paula Bernard Craig
Susan Marie Croteau
Deborah Frances Dueger
Catherine Emery Fernandez
Deborah Lacey Gagnon
Georgette Rita Gagnon
Cynthia Sawyer Langevin
Doreen Lucille Levesque

Sandra Louise MacDonald
Joyce Ladurantaye Saturley
Marlene Sandra Seaman
Evelyn Rogers Sheehy
Cheryl Elaine Smith
Darlene Marie Stanley
Linda Anne Steussing
Lois Ann Wheeler
Jane Nauss Williams

1971

Jane Theresa Anderson
Carole Anne Breton
Suzanne Lucienne
    Charpentier
Martha Akerman Flanders
Diane Marie George
Paula Ann Golden
Rebecca Elizabeth Grant
Barbara Gaffney Hixon
Susan Ellen Jamieson
Linda Lee Laqueux
Patricia Louise Lake
Pauline Lorraine LeBlanc
Donna Ruth Lewis
Sharon Burdette Lupien
Elizabeth Beal McMaster
Valerie Ann Narkunas
Sharon Marie Ouimette
Lorraine Antoinette Presby
Karen McNeely Rosi
Cynthia Joyce Salisbury
Patricia Sweeney Sargent
Joyce Ann Towsley
Linda Karen Trites
Carol Isabel Welch
Bonnie Lee Woodbury

1972

Janice Karen Bresell
Jane Louise Collins
Holly McKeith DeGroot
Teresa Ann Drake
Elaine Diane Drobysh
Lynn Jeanette Farnham
Susan Theresa Ferland
Ann Marie Gallant
Martha Estelle Gerry
Mary Jane Gilbert
Shirley Ellen Hollis
Nancy Ann Isham
Sarah Ann Janik
Pauline Noel Johansen

Ann Marie Langevin
Louise Laurette Langevin
Patricia Arthura Launay
Carol Susan Lavoie
Donna Jean Morrison
Cynthia Jane Petell
Bette Ann Philibert
Barbara Jean Reinhart
Pamela Gray Savard
Mary Lou Shabbott
Corrine Dubel Shannon
Jeannette Karen Skidmore
Linda Katherine Vincent
Holly Gaige Wentworth
Deanna Rose Woodward

1973

Lenny Lee Bennett
Marla Eve Bragdon
Patricia Louise Collins
Carol Ann Flamand
Susan Chappell Frysinger
Bette Anne Gard
Monique Claire Gauthier
Judith Marie Huckins
Patricia Daly Jones
Susan Patricia Knight
Linda Mae Lepene
Denise Laurette Neveu
Deborah Leigh Phillips
Ronda Frances Piro
Sandra Jean Santone
Kathleen Elizabeth Swan
Judith Lorraine Topple
Kay Lois Willis
Jane Lorelei Wilson
Sandra Lee Woodrow

1974

Gertrude Gagnon Alley
Debra Anne Beamish
Esther Lindsay Bettez
Kristel Barbara Brochu
Susan Leslie Claar
Donna Jean Collins
Juanita Edith Durgin
Holly Hall Emerson
Dana Elizabeth Farnum
Susan Marie Geoffroy
Andrea Wheaton Graffam
Theresa Ann Guay
Kathleen Ruth Helms
Deborah Nancy Johnson

Anne Marie LaVoice
Madeleine Doris Leclerc
Candice Ann Leonard
Sandra Kenison McCormack
Margaret Edna Pelletier
Bonnie Lee Shortt
Anne Elizabeth Smith
Claire Gallant Toner
Linda Hurd Tuttle
Patti May Vosburgh
Julianne Whitney Warren

1975

Holly Elizabeth Aebischer
Colleen Mae Annis
Carol Jean Blake
Diana Marie Bowley
Diane Rachel Carrier
Susan Elaine Clark
Debra Louise Cross
Donna Tankard Gagne
Geralyn Anne Gagne
Deborah Bowie Gosselin
Martha Jane Hanson
Dorothy Frances Jewell
Denise Marie Lavoie
Michelle Therese Levesque
Sandra Ann Lucas
Wendy Mae Martin
Alice Marie McDonald
Christie Jean McGreevy
Roxanne Lucille Miville
Linda Denise Moreau
Brenda Stevens Morse
Dolores Esther Robbins
Leslie Carol Salisbury
Patricia Lavoie Sanborn
Debra Savoy Sawyer
Elizabeth Muriel Shorette
Linda Jean Small
Sheila Ann Strout
Denise Allyn Sullivan
June Leslie Tallarico
Denise Marie Turmelle
Mary Jane Willett
Sandra Grondin Wilson
Patricia Jean Wright

1976

Anita Louise Belanger
Yvonne Rachel Bergeron
Debra Ann Berntsen
Nancy Lee Biathrow

Pauline Annette Bourbeau
Cynthia Ann Brill
William Michael Brothers
Linda Darlene Carter
Diane Louise Chabot
Sarah Kenney Connor
Eileen Burdette Corbett
Dawn Ann Curtis
Janice Reed Dawson
Sharon Ann Dolloph
Susanne Theresa Filteau
Kenneth Paul Forcier
Lynn Anne Gauthier
Allison Beth Gillchrest
Carol Jean Higgins
Deborah Jean King
Jeanne Emma Lauziere
Janine Lise Leveille
Sharon Ann Lizotte
Marjorie Susan MacGown
Catherine Diana Major
Dolores Marie Marron
Dale Carolyn Morrill
Glenda Nelson Morrissey
Tina Donahue Nadeau
Brenda Louise Noyes
Nancy Lee Richer
Judith Anne Ross
Betty Lou Ryan
Margot Hammond Saurwein
Cheryl Stevens
Cynthia Ann Stevens
Janet Elizabeth Tousley
Sue Kathryn Weston
Catherine Anne Wiles
Kristine Joan Wilson

1977

Elaine Marie Bertrand
Nancy Leigh Carr
Gail Higgins Cayer
Bonnie Lee Chase
Paula Binette Chouinard
Paullette Theresa Croteau
Diane Davis
Susan Patricia Debelis
Kimberly Ann Engelsen
Mary Ellen Erb
Laurette Anne Grenier
Marjorie Marie Hadlock
Lisa Marie Hardy
Susan Beth Hendrick

Jocelyn Gail Hunter
Paula Jane LaClair
Patricia Ann Levesque
Sharon Poluchov Lincoln
Ann Cleaves Lorden
Marcia Dixwell Moore
Marilyn Jane Morse
Arthur Joseph Nadeau
Denise Elaine Nadeau
Debra Ann Nelson
Bonnie Ann Nicoletti
Kathleen Monique Page
Isabel Maria Peixinho
Sally Fay Rogers
Faith Irene Sanderson
Deborah Ellen Swasey
Linda Geralyn Tetreault
Lauren Marie Trombley
Karen Rose Trostle
Diane Holl Tyrrel

1978

Callie Ann Atkins
Sandra Sims Avallone
Anne Ferman Beaudoin
Cheryl Anne Bronson
Jean Cassady Dineen
Cathleen Gilchrist Donohue
Karen June Foster
Debra Elaine Franks
Catherine Gaffney
Susan Diane Haines
Debra Ann Hallyburton
Donna Marie Hilliard
Nancy Kavalauskas
Patti Shabbott Koscielniak
Theresa Irene Lemire
Jan Marie Levesque
Jo-Ellen Anita Lewis
Elizabeth Patricia Manners
Susan Marie Mayhew
Frances Gilroy Moline
Beverly Wellman
  Moscaritolo
E. Jane O'Connor
Lisa Marie Ramsay
Colleen Jaye Rutherford
Linda Ayers Severance
Kathryn Joy Smith
Donna Lee Tonkin
Roberta Maxine Tuttle
Madeleine Boucher
  Vaillancourt

A Kindly Interest

1979

Betty Gayle Batcha
Sharon Lee Bennett
Catherine Anne Bilodeau
Karen Ann Boothroyd
Robert James Buchholtz
Teresa Jane Byron
Susan Marie Carrier
Vicki Ann Cookson
Roxanne Smith Cowley
Tyyne Estella Cox
Althea Rose Drew
Kathleen Ann Dunn
Cindy Flora Forcier
Mary Ellen Hanley
Candace Louise Jacques
Roxanne Joy
Paula Anita Labonte
Anne Irene Latva
Yolanda Ruth Leal
Lori Littlefield
Jane Louise Lombardi
Susan Gracie MacLeod
Janet Ann Noyes
Susan Podziewski Olivier
Lucille Pauline Poulin
Margaret Lynn Richards
Denise Marie Roy
Jerrilyn Blackwell Sargent
Jane Lucette Schinella
Donna Marie Scott
Marybeth Shutt Snow
Susan Thorsen Still
Susan Rita Thibeault
Roberta H. Waldron
Marie Jane White
Cynthia Louise Young

1980

Louise Aline Bourque
Laura Lee Bowler
Michelle Mae Chapin
Beverly Jean Dalphond
Karen Lee Davis
Cheryl Ann Edwards
Irene Semolic Hanslin
Pamela Jean Horne
Mary Katherine Iacopino
Susan Pearl Lambert
Jacqueline Ann Landry
Kelly Jean Loisel
Kim Susan Martell

Gaye Catherine Martin
Cynthia Carolyn McDonald
Sharon May McIntire
Vicki Lynn McLain
Teresa May Moulton
Pamela Ann Olivier
Wanda Cummiford Osborne
Mary Palmer
Elizabeth Hamlin Perkins
Andrea Polachek
Tammy Anne Riley
Carol Lynn Robinson
Rachelle Denise Roy
Margaret Lenore Schaffnit
Colleen Croteau Tewksbury
Margaret Edith Wareing
Mary Elizabeth Welch

1981

Donna Ross Allard
Susan Mildred Allin
Ramona Pearl Anderson
Patti Ann Angers
Irene St. Gelais Arnold
Tracey Caldwell Bergeron
Donna Lee Bonneau
Lisa Zotto Borden
Linda Christine Charest
Janet Elizabeth Coughlin
Karen Jeannette Davis
Joan Irene Delisle
Dawn Judith Drouin
Lisa Marie Dumont
Lorri Lynn Fluet
Sandra Lee Harper
Raye-Jean Higgins
Paul Hopwood
Deborah Gail Irish
Ruth English Keith
Noel Marie LaClair
Janet Marie Lacroix
Debra Ann Lariviere
Rebecca Allen Millimet
Michelle Ann Ouellette
Lynda Vee Patrick
Sharon Lee Patton
Linda Susan Prescott
Debra Ruth Smith
Pamela Jane Venner
Kimberly Ellen Vitale
Wayne A. Weeks, Jr.

1982

Beverly Jean Bartlett
Rena Ann Blackburn
Aimee Marie Brownell
Mary Ann Chorlton
Douglas Gene Cushman
Laurie Ann Erickson
Heidi Ann Gerhard
Monica Ann Gilman
Joyce Ellen Kingsbury
Jody Sherman Martin
Susan McCrosky
Sheila McCabe Mitchell
Lu Ann Moody
Patricia Mary Ann
  Allen Patz
Debra E. Preston
Leah Anne Roy
Michelle Arlene Roy
Beth Marie Smith
Ruth Ada Twombly
Kathy Lynn Urquhart

1983

Laurie Faye Belhumeur
Gina Louise Bibbo
Ellen Louise Bishop
Elizabeth Ellen Bouley
Linda Sue Bowersox
Diane Lynda Chevalier
Theresa Lynn Cote
Cindy Louise Cox
Dena Marie Demarais
Leanne Marie Downing
Robin Marcelle Downs
Mary Ellen Durant
Diane Marie Forest
Mary Ellen Fournier
Elaine Rogers Gonyo
Dorothy Ann Hook
Michelle Anne Jean
Pamela Madden Laflamme
Shari Lynn Laurion
Carol Allison Lebold
Christine Fay Parratt
Marjorie Ann Raible
Karen Elizabeth Ramus
Charlene Elaine Reynolds
Linda Ann St. Hilaire
Vivian Claire Sweeney
Roslyn Marie Todd

1984

Michelle Jacqueline
  Anderson
Jennifer Bede
Nadine Rose Boucher
Lynne Ann Chambers
Patricia Verne Coughlin
Sandra Lee Croteau
Diane Marie Dumont
Maria Preston Ellis
Karen Lee Glidden
Beverly Daigle Grappone
Francene Elaine Huot
Tammy Sue Kiniry
Lee Ann Bailey Lavoie
Joyce MacIntosh
Sheryl Irene Pastene
Nancy Elizabeth Perkins
Christine Ann Racette
Ruth Ann Rehm
Donna Lyn Remillard
Joanne Irene Roy
Victoria Janet Ryan
Sharon Wiley Scott
Teresa Scoville
Marie Juneau Simpson
Lori Ann Sloane
Dana Lynne Thayer
Suzanne Marthe Valcour

1985

Donna Ree Allen
Cindy Ridge Baudendistel
Cynthia Anne Boivin
Patricia Lee Collins
Deborah Anne Dorley
Theresa Marie Fournier
JoAnn Lisa Garceau
Lisa Lilly Houle
Lisa Kendrick
Kathleen Louise Koch
Catherine Ann Michaels
Deborah Jean Montgomery
Elizabeth Fay Moore
Denise Ellen Morin
Deborah Jane Oscroft

Patricia Antoinette Perkins
Margaret Brigid Quinn
Elizabeth Leorah Rodgers
Laurie Ann Rogers
Michele Ann Roseberry
Elizabeth Jane Sibson
Cynthia Lindsey Tuttle
Jo Ann Warnke
Jo Ann Wentworth

1986

Karen Jane Ballou
Michelle Anne Beaupre
Karen Marie Bennett
Susan Culbertson Brighton
Christine Lorette Chickering
Penny Jane Clattenburg
Laurel Ann Corson
Linda Claire Duquette
Jane Louise Eaton
Lisa Marie Ellis
Karen Marie Faucette
Christine Ann Fournier
Lori Anne Gray
Nathan Arnold Hersom
Roberta Charlotte Hiltz
Gregory Clark Jenkins
Cynthia Joyce Jenness
Karen Sue Laventure
Michele Therese Melanson
Jennifer Anne Norsworthy
Shelly Ann O'Brien
Laura Mae Ruths
Brien Keith Stanley

1987

Melissa Irene Bennett
Julie Ann Bowen
Wendy Sue Carney
Judy Ann Gilbert
Pamela Jane Gould
Cheryl Florence Hilliard
Deborah Jane Lortz
Karen Marie Meagher
Sharon Alice Meserve
Lynn Louise Moyer

Cynthia Ann Shappell
Ann Tracy Stokes
Colleen Ann Weeks
Lorelee Ann Wetherbee

1988

Linda Lee Artz
Deborah Anne Bernier
Hannah Marie Boisvert
Linda Aline Brooks
Laurie Ann Cailler
Caron B. Cohn
Marjorie Paige DuBois
Jane Ann Durkin
Nora Durning
Robin Fletcher Dwane
Joann E. Harrison
Jacqueline Hernon
Kimberly Houle Jewell
Christine Allison Kalway
Tina Carla Laurentz
Rachel Theresa L'Heureux
Heather Ann Livingston
Nancy Claudette Marquis
Joan Elizabeth Matthews
Cathy Lynn Ordway
Lisa Marie Piet
Michelle Ann Piurkowski
Cheryl Annette Price
Thomas Henry Raymond
Judith Olson Rossiter
Robin Jean Sanborn
Joanne Marie Therrien
Carol Anne Wilson
Tricia Anne Wormwood

1989

Collette Ann Beaulieu
Josephine White Boyce
Tracy Ann Campbell
Diana Lynn Focht
Kathleen Elaine Kenney
Nancy Ann Leedberg
Pamela Ray Paris
Tina Marie St. Pierre
Teresa Anne Welch

A Kindly Interest

Sample Curricula

Class of 1930
New Hampshire Memorial Hospital School of Nursing
Summary of Program*
Length of program 3 years

Year	Term or Semester	Course	Total Hours or Credits of Instruction	Total Days of Practice
1,2		Anatomy & Physiology	55	
1,2		Applied Bacteriology & Pathology	30	
1		Personal Hygiene	18	
		Nutrition & Cookery; Dietetics	36	61
		Drugs & Solutions	22	
		Elementary Nursing	60	62
		History & Social Aspects of Nursing	15	
		Materia Medica & Therapeutics	40	
		Elementary Principles of Massage	12	
		Ethics	15	
2		Nursing in General Medical Diseases	15	248
		Surgical & Gynecological Nursing	15	221
		Pediatric Nursing	15	204
		Obstetrical Nursing	10	213
		Nervous & Mental Nursing	8	
		Modern Social Conditions	9	
3		Nursing in Communicable Diseases	12	61
		Total	387	1070

Institutions and agencies used for
learning experiences by the School of
Nursing: Belmont Hospital of City of
Worcester Health Department,
Worcester, Mass.

*Sample Plan as instruction hours and
clinical days varied by student.

Class of 1953
Concord Hospital School of Nursing
Summary of Program*
Length of program 3 years

Year	Term or Semester	Course	Total Hours or Credits of Instruction	Total Days of Practice
1		Anatomy & Physiology	117	
		Chemistry	57	
		Microbiology	51	
		Psychology	31	
		Sociology	30	
		Pharmacology	60	
		History of Nursing	30	
		Foods & Nutrition	45	
		Diet Therapy	20	42
		Intr. to Medical Science	31	
		Social Problems in Nursing	17	
		Nursing	301	
		Medical-Surgical Nursing	154	283
		Operating Room Nursing	30	104
		Emergency Nursing	20	
1,2,3		Professional Adjustments	51	
2		Communicable Disease Nursing	27	
		Dermatological Nursing	14	
		Eye, Ear, Nose, Throat Nursing	28	18
		Gynecological Nursing	19	31
		Orthopedic Nursing	17	37
		Urological Nursing	17	23
		Dentistry	5	
		Obstetric Nursing	67	61
		Nursing of Newborn		30
3		Tuberculosis Nursing	62	61
		Nursing of Children	106	54
		Formula Room		8
		Psychiatric Nursing	160	92
		Nursing & Health Service in the Family	15	
		Outpatient Nursing		14
		Total	1582	858

Institutions and agencies used for learning experiences by the School of Nursing: The Children's Hospital, Columbus, Ohio; Benjamin Franklin Hospital, Columbus, Ohio; N.H. State Hospital, Concord, New Hampshire.

*Sample Plan as clinical days varied by student.

A Kindly Interest

Class of 1971
Concord Hospital School of Nursing
Summary of Program
Length of program 133 weeks*

Year	Term or Semester	Course	Total Hours or Credits of Instruction	Total Hours of Practice
1	1	Microbiology	45	
1	1	Sociology	30	
1	1	Anatomy and Physiology	93	
1	1	Psychology	72	
1	1	Chemistry	64	
1	1	Nutrition	24	
1	1	Fundamentals of Nursing	117	56
1	2	Care of the Adult Medical-Surgical Patient Part I	132	228
1	3	Care of the Adult Medical-Surgical Patient Part II	132	228
2	1	Care of the Adult Medical-Surgical Patient Part III	136	228
2	2	Care of the Patient Requiring Surgery	108	312
2	3	Nursing of Children	96	274
2	4	Maternity Nursing	96	324
3	1	Psychiatric & Mental Health Nursing	137	282
3	2	Care of the Adult Medical-Surgical Patient Part IV	102	245
3	2	Professional Responsibilities & Opportunities	24	
3	3	Introduction to Team Leadership	66	336
		Total	1474	2513

*When pertinent, include theory and related practice as one course. † If practice is recorded in hours, change column heading.

Institutions and agencies used for learning experiences by the School of Nursing: New Hampshire Hospital, Concord, New Hampshire; The Children's Hospital Medical Center, Boston, Massachusetts.

*Terms: 1st year - 1-24 weeks and 2-12 weeks
2nd year - 4-12 weeks
3rd year - 3-12 weeks

Class of 1989
Concord Hospital School of Nursing
Summary of Program
Length of program 112 weeks*

Year	Term or Semester	Course	Total Hours or Credits of Instruction	Total Hours of Practice
1	1	Psyc 401-Intro to Psychology*	4 cr.	
	1	Biol 305-Medical Microbiology & Lab*	4 cr.	
	1	Biol 211-Human Anatomy & Physiology I*	3 cr.	
	1	Biol 213-Human Anatomy & Physiology I Lab*	1 cr.	
	1	Nursing 101-Fundamentals of Nursing	90	45
1	2	Soso 551-Human Development*	4 cr.	
	2	Nut 448-Normal & Therapeutic Nutrition*	4 cr.	
	2	Biol 212-Human Anatomy & Physiology II*	3 cr.	
	2	Biol 214-Human Anatomy & Physiology II Lab*	1 cr.	
	2	Nursing 102-Fundamentals of Nursing II	75	150
1	3	Nursing 201-Adult Medical Surgical Nursing I	50	150
2	1	Soc 400-Intro to Sociology*	4 cr.	
		Nursing 202-Adult Medical Surgical Nursing II	90	270
	2	Nursing 203-Parent & Child Nursing	105	315
	3	Nursing 205-Adult Medical Surgical Nursing III	50	150
3	1	Nursing 204-Psychiatric & Surgical Nursing	105	315
	2	Nursing Trends	15	
	2	Nursing 301-Advanced Nursing	90	360
			29 cr. +	
		Total	670 hrs.	1755

Institutions and agencies used for
learning experiences by the School of
Nursing: School for Lifelong Learning
- University System of N.H.

*Terms 1 and 2 of each year - 16 weeks
Term 3, Year 1 and 2 - 8 weeks

Notes

Where sources are not given they are from the bound volumes of the boards of trustees of the three hospitals, beginning with July 1884. Extensive use was made of *Concord Monitor* articles, the earliest from bound volumes at the Concord Public Library, later from scrapbooks kept by the hospitals. The School of Nursing's records were consulted. Historical materials were solicited of nursing school alumni and of hospital employees. The author had nearly a dozen interviews and informal conversations with individuals which illuminated the past and defined the present.

Chapter 1

1. *Concord Monitor,* January 2, 1884.
2. *Ibid.,* January 29, 1884.
3. Lyford, James O., ed., *History of New Hampshire, 1854-1902,* v. 2, p. 1066.
4. *American Heritage Pictorial History of the Presidents of the United States.* American Heritage Publishing Company, 1968, pp. 550-51, 659.
5. Lyford, p. 907.
6. Kalisch, Philip A. and Beatrice J., *The Advance of American Nursing.* Little, Brown and Company, Boston, 1978, p. 23.
7. *Ibid.,* pp. 33-42.
8. *Ibid.,* p. 44.
9. *Nursing Research,* Reverby, Susan, "Womanhood and Nursing in Historical Perspective," v. 36, no. 1, January-February, 1987, pp. 5-10.
10. *Ibid.,* pp. 5-10.
11. Dolan, Josephine, A., *Nursing in Society.* W.B. Saunders Company, Philadelphia, 1973, p. 194.
12. Kalisch, p. 88.

Chapter 2

1. Bouton, Nathaniel, *History of Concord, 1725-1853.* Benning W. Sanborn, Concord, 1856, p.440.
2. Bouton, p. 573.
3. Dolan, p. 193.
4. Kalisch, pp. 81-2.
5. Lyford, p. 950.
6. Streeter, Lilian Carpenter, letter to Mrs. Maude D. Emmons, trustee, Margaret Pillsbury Hospital, October 24, 1934.

7. Lyford, p. 951.
8. *Ibid.,* pp. 952-5.
9. Unidentified publication, appendix, pp. 47-108 describing dedication of Margaret Pillsbury Hospital.

Chapter 3

1. Streeter letter.
2. *Concord Monitor,* March 21, 1890.
3. *Ibid.,* March 21, 1890.
4. *Ibid.,* March 22, 1890.
5. Lyford, pp. 952-5.
6. Kalisch, pp. 109-12.
7. Annual Report of the Margaret Pillsbury Hospital, 1934.

Chapter 4

1. Reprint from *Medical Woman's Journal,* October, 1928, unpaged, Wallace, Ellen A., MD, "The New Hampshire Memorial Hospital for Women and Children."
2. Articles of Association and Constitution of the Women's Hospital Aid Association, Concord, 1896.
3. Lyford, p. 957.
4. Kalisch, p. 134.
5. *Ibid.,* pp. 155-60.
6. Handwritten report of Laura Meader to board of trustees, Margaret Pillsbury Hospital, April 1, 1917.
7. Actually, the journal *Trained Nurse* preceded *AJN,* its first issues dating back to the 1880s. It later became *Trained Nurse and Hospital Review.*

Chapter 5

1. John Pearson, a wealthy Concord businessman left an estate in trust for charitable purposes at his death in 1899. One of the oldest in New Hampshire it was administered by three trustees until 1980 when its assets were absorbed into the unrestricted funds of the New Hampshire Charitable Fund.

2. Kalisch, pp. 259-62.

3. New Hampshire Board of Nursing, "Outline of Developments in Nursing Through Legislation in New Hampshire," 1975.

4. Kalisch, pp. 265-7.

5. *Ibid.*, pp. 289-90.

6. Brittain, Vera, *Testament of Youth*, Seaview Books, New York, 1980.

7. Annual Report, Margaret Pillsbury General Hospital, 1918.

8. *Ibid.*, 1934.

9. *Concord Monitor*, November 11, 1918. (advertisement).

Chapter 6

1. Annual Report, Margaret Pillsbury General Hospital, 1934.

2. *Concord Monitor*, September 7, 1921.

3. *New Hampshire Notables*, Concord Press, 1932.

4. *Ibid.*

5. Langley, James M., et al, "Report of the Committee of Nine." New Hampshire Memorial Hospital, Concord, 1938.

6. *Concord Monitor*, December 12, 1936.

Chapter 7

1. Annual Report, Margaret Pillsbury General Hospital, 1934. Years later another Pillsbury graduate, Cora Sweatt (Gray), 1943, became known as the "Angel of Unalaska" for her ministrations to the population of a small Aleutian island. She retired after forty-six years as a nurse in 1969.

2. Letter to School of Nursing from Ruth Inman (Tozier), Fall, 1986.

3. Letter to author from Genevieve Mullen (McDonald), April 9, 1987.

4. Abbie Emmons, conversation with the author, September 9, 1988.

5. Stern, Jane and Michael, *Square Meals*. Alfred Knopf, New York, 1984, pp. 198-245. Sometime during 1949, the nursing school and alumnae brought out their own 315-page cookbook, *Concord Cuisine*, which contains recipes in the handwriting of their contributors and handdrawn ads for local businesses.

6. Kalisch, pp. 473-5.

Chapter 8

1. *New Hampshire Notables, 1932*. Additional information on Langley found in obituary written by him for *Concord Monitor*, June 24, 1968.

2. The incorporators were, in addition to Langley, Couch and Duncan: Robert W. Potter, Gardner Tilton, I. Reed Gourley, Douglas N. Everett, Charlotte N. Brooks, Fanny S. Lake, Emma A. Knapp, Helen H. Brunel, Mrs. A.B. Presby, Patrick J. Bolger, Harry G. Emmons, Harold H. Blake, J. Mitchell Ahern, Roy W. Peaslee, Ray W. Pert, Edgar C. Hirst, Ruth Fernald Holst, Helen G. Pelren, Amoret N. Hollis, Gladys B. Dolloff, Martha J. Nelson, Frank J. Sulloway, Walter C. Jenkins, Frank McSwiney.

3. The city discovered in the early seventies that there were two Grandviews, the other being Grandview Road in Bow. To prevent confusion the street adjoining the hospital's property became Rum Hill Road, honoring the old name for the hill.

Chapter 9

1. The New Concord Hospital, Concord Hospital Building Fund, 1946.

2. *The Valley Times*, Lebanon, New Hampshire, November 8, 1946.

3. *Concord Monitor*, February 8, 1947.

4. *Ibid.*

5. Angus M. Brooks, conversation with the author, October 1988.

6. Letter from James M. Langley to Concord Hospital Board of Trustees, December 18, 1950.

7. *Concord Monitor*, January 5, 1953.

8. *Ibid.*, September 27, 1951.

9. *Ibid.*, December 17, 1952.

10. *Ibid.*, May 5, 1953.

11. *Ibid.*, April 8, 1953.

12. Norman R. Brown, conversation with the author, October 15, 1988.

Chapter 10

1. *Life Lines*, Concord Hospital, v. 8, no. 2, Spring, 1988.

2. Pamphlet on dedication of Concord Hospital, April 14, 1956.

3. Langley's displeasure with the final plans for the nursing school building was evident to those who stood near him at its dedication when he was overheard to say, "I dedicate this the backhouse."

4. Patricia Tobin, conversation with the author, Spring, 1987.

5. Harper, James Jr., The Life of Leonhard Felix Fuld. Marine Midland Bank, Investment Services Division, New York, 1969.

6. Report of the Concord Area Health Survey, 1980.

7. Letter from Oliver Fifield to Board of Trustees, Concord Hospital, April 4, 1980.

8. Richard Fredrickson, Concord Hospital treasurer, is responsible for sorting out the complexities of the reorganization.

9. Interview with Marjorie DuBois, class of 1988, Concord Hospital School of Nursing, March 1988.

Bibliography

Books, Periodicals and Reports

The American Heritage Pictorial History of the Presidents of the United States, v. 2. American Heritage Publishing Company, 1968.

American Journal of Nursing, special section, "Nurses for the Future," v. 87, no. 12, pp. 1593-1648.

Bouton, Nathaniel, *The History of Concord, 1725-1853*. Benning W. Sanborn, Concord, 1856.

Brittain, Vera, *Testament of Youth*. Seaview Books, New York, 1980.

Bullough, Vern L. and Bonnie, *History, Trends and Politics of Nursing*. Appleton-Century-Crofts, Norwalk, Connecticut, 1984.

Dolan, Josephine A., *Nursing in Society*. W.B. Saunders Company, Philadelphia, 1973.

Godey's Lady's Book and Magazine, v. 86, January-June, 1873.

Goostray, Stella, *Memoirs: Half a Century in Nursing*. Nursing Archive, Boston University Mugar Library, The Reporter Press, North Conway, New Hampshire, 1969.

Harper, James, Jr., The Life of Leonhard Felix Fuld. Marine Midland Bank Investment Services Division, New York, 1969.

Helene Fuld Health Trust, Annual Reports. Marine Midland Bank, New York, 1977, 1982-83, 1987.

Kalisch, Philip A. and Beatrice J., *The Advance of American Nursing*. Little, Brown and Company, Boston, 1978.

Lyford, James O., ed., *History of Concord 1854-1902*, v. 2, Concord, 1903.

Metcalf, Henry N., Abbott, Frances, *1000 New Hampshire Notables*. Rumford Printing Company, Concord, 1919.

New Hampshire Board of Nursing Education and Nurse Registration, "Laws of New Hampshire Relating to Professional and Practical Nurses." Concord, 1982.

New Hampshire Charitable Fund and Affiliated Trusts, Annual Reports. Concord, 1980, 1987.

New Hampshire Notables. Concord Press, Concord, 1932.

New Hampshire State Board of Nurse Examiners, "Registration of Nurses." Concord, 1944.

New Hampshire State Board of Nursing, "Outline of Developments in Nursing Through Legislation in New Hampshire." Concord, 1975.

New Hampshire State Board of Nursing Education and Nurse Registration, "Summary of Legislation of Nursing in New Hampshire." Concord, 1973.

Nightingale, Florence, *Notes on Nursing: What It Is And What It Is Not*, (facsimile ed. of original). Harrison, London, 1859, pub. by J.B. Lippincott Company, Philadelphia, 1946.

Nursing Research, Reverby, Susan, "A Caring Dilemma: Womanhood and Nursing in Historical Perspective," v. 36, no. 1, January-February, 1987.

Report of the Concord Area Health Survey, Concord, 1980.

Reverby, Susan, *Ordered to Care*. Cambridge University Press, Cambridge Press, New York, 1987.

Richards, Linda, *Reminiscences of Linda Richards, America's First Trained Nurse*. Whitcomb and Barrows, Boston, 1915.

Rosenberg, Charles E., *The Care of Strangers*. Basic Books, Inc., New York, 1987.

Stern, Jane and Michael, *Square Meals*. Alfred Knopf, New York, 1984.

Winant, John G., *Letter from Grovesnor Square*. Houghton Mifflin Company, Boston, 1947.

Wise, P.M., *A Text-Book for Training Schools for Nurses*, v. 2. G.P. Putnam's Sons, New York, 1897.

Hospital and School of Nursing Publications

Appendix to unidentified publication pp. 47-108, dedication of the Margaret Pillsbury Hospital, October 1891.

Articles of Association and Constitution of the Women's Hospital Aid Association, Concord, New Hampshire, 1896.

Breene, Dorothy M., et al, *New Hampshire Hospital Historical Highlights*. Alumni Association of the New Hampshire Hospital School of Nursing, Taylor Publishing Company, 1983.

"Caring," Concord Hospital Expansion Fund, Concord, 1980.

"Commemorative Opportunities and Living Tributes," Concord Hospital Expansion Fund, 1980.

Concord Cuisine, Concord Hospital School of Nursing, 1949.

Concord Hospital, Annual Reports: 1969, 1972-75, 1977-87.

Concord Hospital School of Nursing Closing Report to the National League for Nursing, Concord, March 1988.

Concord Hospital School of Nursing Self-Evaluation Report to the New Hampshire Board of Nursing, Concord, 1985.

Concord Hospital School of Nursing yearbooks: *The Nutrix*, 1951-54, 1956, 1964, 1969. Untitled, 1976, 1983-84, 1987.

Concord Monitor, special section, "Concord Hospital Dedication of the New Hospital Addition," May 15, 1982.

Langley, James M., et al, "Report of the Committee of Nine," New Hampshire Memorial Hospital, Concord, 1938.

Life Lines, Concord Hospital, v. 8, no. 2, Spring 1988.

Margaret Pillsbury General Hospital, Annual Reports, Concord, 1918-21, 1923-25, 1929, 1933, 1935-40, 1942-44.

Margaret Pillsbury Training School yearbook, *Vigilance*, 1943.

"The New Concord Hospital," Concord Hospital Building Fund, 1946.

New Hampshire Memorial Hospital Annual Report, Concord, 1943.

Illustrations and Credits

With two exceptions, all the illustrations in this volume were selected from the archives of the Concord Hospital. The photograph of James Langley on page 60 was supplied by the *Concord Monitor* and the early view of the Concord railroad station on page 35 by the New Hampshire Historical Society. The author and publishers are deeply grateful to both for their cooperation. In the following list the photographer's or delineator's name when known appears between the abbreviated caption and the number of the page on which the illustration appears.

Index

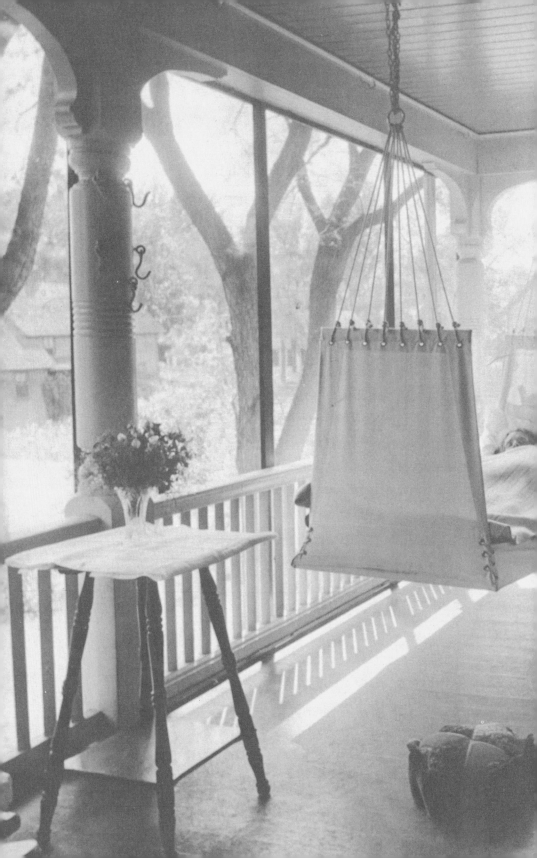